Chapter One

Tools of the Trade

The number and variety of cosmetic products and tools on the market is almost infinite. This means that choosing the right textures, colours and formulations can be a daunting task which often results in expensive trial and error.

Skin tone and texture, eye colour and face shape all come into play when choosing products and brushes, but so too does personal preference. Some makeup artists swear by the crispness of liquid eyeliner, for example, while others grab a gel liner and a flat brush for better control. By getting a feel for the breadth of formulations and colours available – and the strengths and weaknesses of each – you can start to build your own bespoke kit.

While all professionals have a colossal collection of every shade they'll ever need, they will also trim it down to a mobile kit of their favourite fall-backs to carry backstage or on shoots. By investing in some quality skincare, a great primer, base, blush and just a handful of brushes, you'll have a capsule kit to build on. Then you can go wild with the less pricey statement eye and lip products that are led by seasonal trends and colours.

Skincare

1. PRECLEANSE

An optional step in your routine, precleansers are great for cutting through oils, makeup and sunscreens to make the cleansing that follows much more effective. Pro MUAs love this double-cleanse technique as it creates really clean skin as a base.

2. CLEANSER

Cream cleansers are massaged into the skin then removed with a hot cloth, while cleansing milks are applied with a cotton pad. Both methods are great for drier skin types. Water-based cleansers such as micellar water soaked into a cotton pad are quick to use, but often not as effective at cleansing deep into the pores. Foaming cleansers lather up with water and are great for oilier skins, but they can be drying, so remember to follow with a good moisturizer.

3. TONER

Don't skip this step. Toners can clear excess oil, but they also hydrate and create a clear base for serum and moisturizer. Look for alcohol-free formulas. For oily skin, choose a toner with alpha-hydroxy acids such as salicylic acid. Drier skins will benefit from a hydrating, vitamin-packed toner.

4. SERUM OR FACIAL OIL

This is your treatment product. Use it between toning and moisturizing to effect the change you want to achieve in your skin. You can get serums and oils to help treat anything from sensitivity to fine lines, dehydration or acne. The smaller particles in these formulations allow their active ingredients to penetrate the skin to a deeper level than creams.

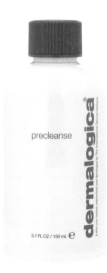
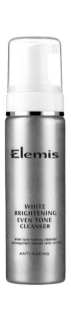
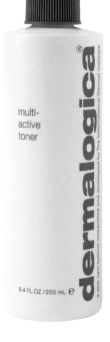
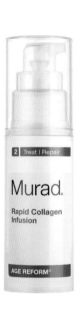
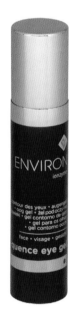
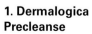

1. Dermalogica Precleanse

2. Elemis White Brightening Cleanser

3. Dermalogica Multi-Active Toner

4. Murad Rapid Collagen Infusion

5. Environ Cquence Eye Gel

It's easy to get set in your ways with makeup, particularly when you're pushed for time in the mornings. This book will encourage you to look at your makeup routine with new enthusiasm. And, while you may not want to channel catwalk trends at work, you can select elements of any of the looks in these pages to enhance your face shape and self-image.

WEARABLE DESIGNS

Just as professional makeup artists translate cutting-edge styles into more wearable designs, keeping on top of makeup trends and experimenting with new styles will help you to widen your repertoire and rediscover your passion for playing with colour and texture. It's also a good idea to update your product picks from time to time as the newest formulations often have advanced active ingredients and staying power not found in older products. In your foundation alone, ditching the full-coverage, matt-finish formula in favour of an illuminating all-day base will instantly update your look, and make application easier in the process.

From the popular 'no-makeup makeup' look to avant garde graphic eyeliner and neon lips, all the styles in this book have been carefully selected to be on-trend but also timeless, so that mastering the techniques behind them will give you skills to reuse and build on for years to come.

As well as breaking down complex techniques into simple step-by-step guides, the later chapters in this book offer a range of inspirational styles. Armed with the knowledge and tools, you can customize them using colours, textures and techniques that best suit your skin, face shape, eye colour, age and, of course, your own personal style.

A metallic eye look by makeup artist Abbi-Rose Crook for a cover shoot for *Professional Beauty* magazine

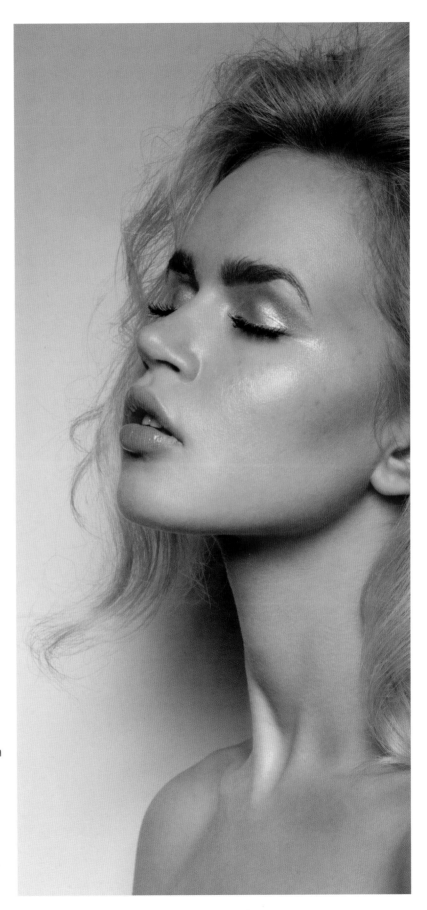

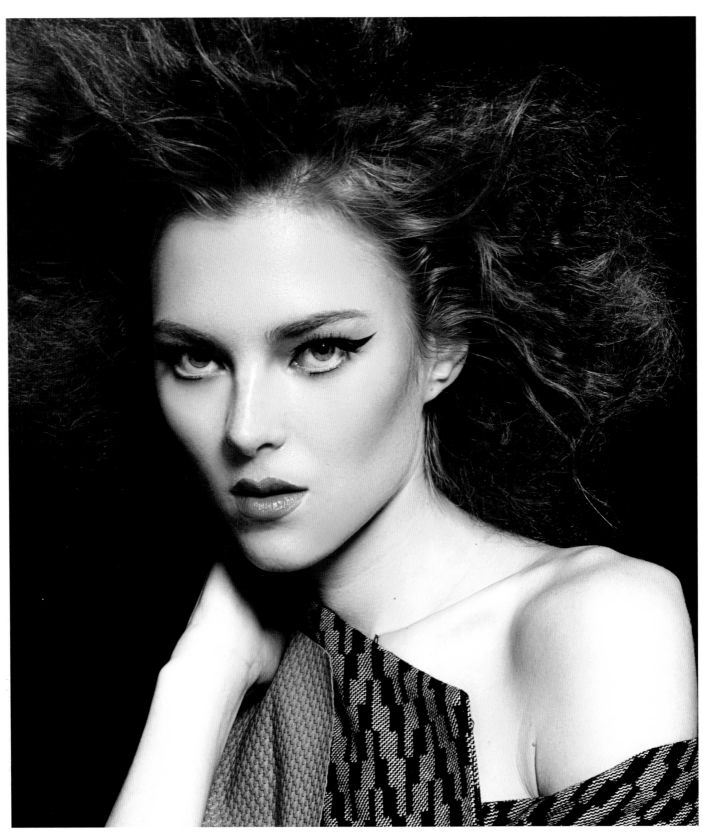

A high-impact look by pro makeup artist Tamara Tott

MAKEUP

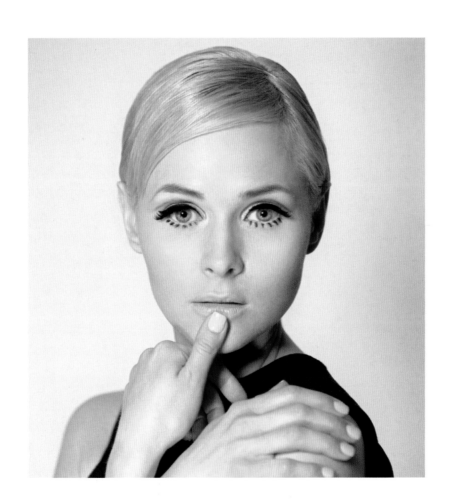

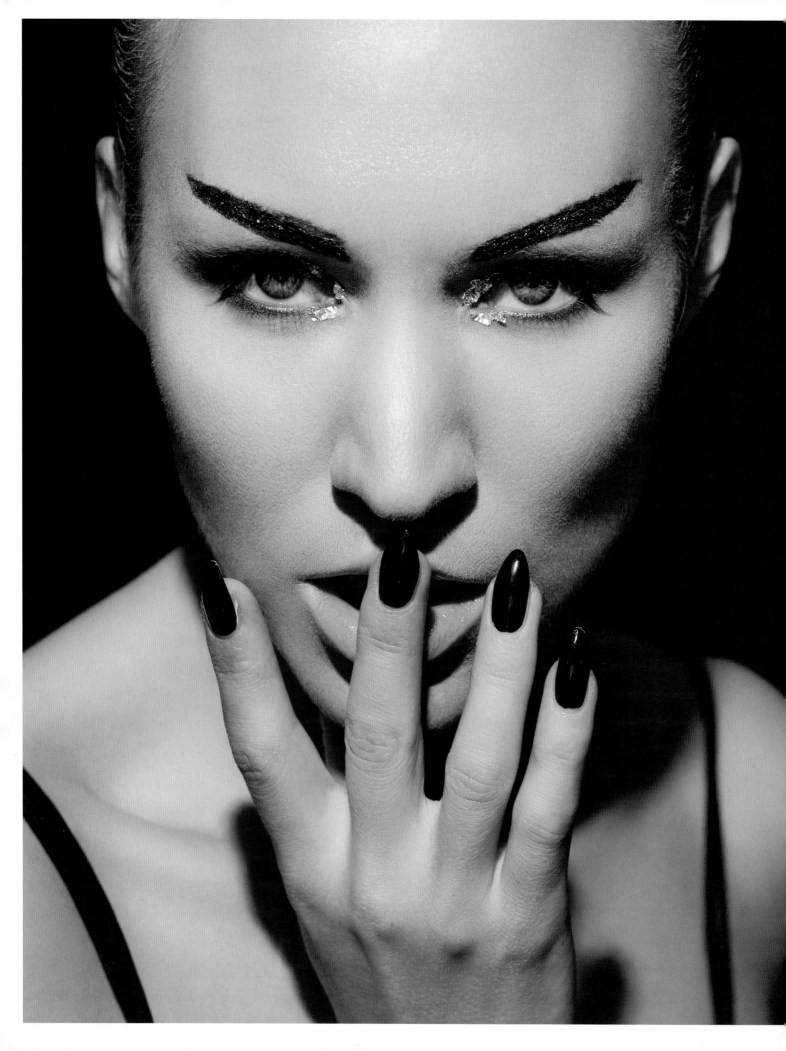

MAKEUP

THE ULTIMATE STEP-BY-STEP GUIDE TO BEAUTY **EVE OXBERRY**

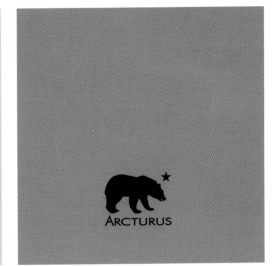

ARCTURUS

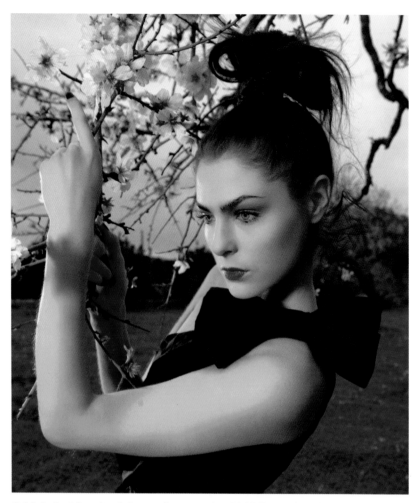

A high-fashion look by makeup artist Abbi-Rose Crook

ARCTURUS

This edition published in 2015 by Arcturus Publishing Limited
26/27 Bickels Yard, 151–153 Bermondsey Street,
London SE1 3HA

ISBN: 978-1-78404-793-1
AD004577UK

Printed in China

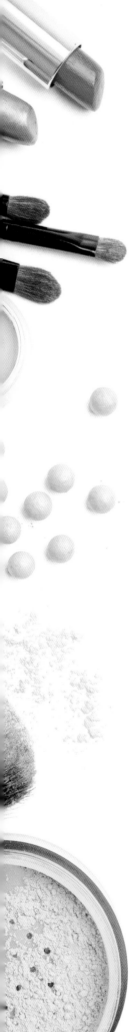

Contents

Introduction

Whether you want to master the perfect red lip or liner flick or simply achieve radiant, glowing skin, there are skills and shortcuts in these pages to help you perfect a professional technique. Unlike the many makeup books already out there, written by a single pro, this guide draws on the talents of some 26 amazing makeup artists to bring you their trade secrets. This way, you can try new techniques and build up a library of skills inspired by a who's who of experts.

All the makeup artists (MUAs) who share their tips over the following pages have vast experience in creating inspirational work for catwalk shows, editorial and campaign shoots, celebrities and demanding brides. When space and time are tight, these women and men know how to deliver, and have some great tricks for cutting down on application time and keeping makeup flawless throughout the pressures of a demanding day.

But beyond all that, they know immediately how to make any woman look fantastic, enhancing her best features to bring out her natural beauty so that it's the face you notice, not the makeup. Makeup is about enhancing what you already have, not changing your appearance. By emphasizing your best features and minimizing those you like less, great makeup skills mean that you still look and feel like yourself – just a more radiant version.

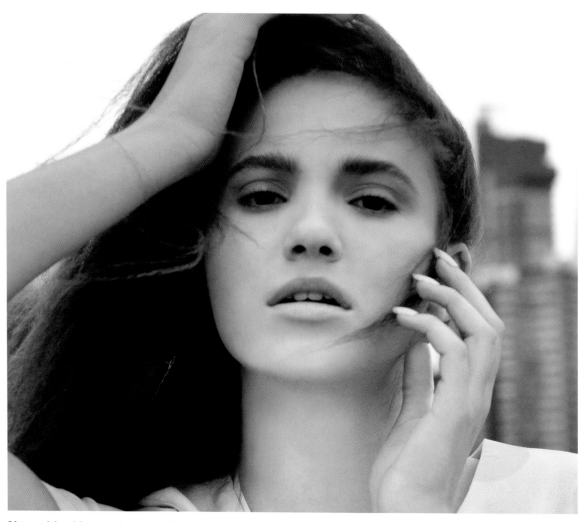

Natural-looking makeup by Melanie Brown for a shoot by Tory Smith

5. EYE CREAM

The skin around your eyes is thinner than elsewhere on the face, so normal moisturizer may be too heavy for this area. Eye creams hydrate and can also treat problems – look out for ingredients such as vitamin C or kojic acid to treat dark circles, caffeine to counteract puffiness, and collagen-boosting peptides to reduce fine lines. Always apply eye cream before moisturizer so that the eye area absorbs only this product.

6. MOISTURIZER

Invest in a light day cream with an SPF and non-greasy finish to apply under makeup. Use a heavier night cream, as your skin repairs itself at night and can take something richer. Try a fluid for summer or hot climates and a thicker cream for winter months.

7. EXFOLIATOR

A weekly essential to slough off dead cells, get the skin glowing and improve absorption. Choose mechanical exfoliation via small beads or grains, or chemical exfoliation via alpha or beta hydroxy acids. These are not as scary as they sound and many come from natural sources such as fruits.

8. MASK

Use a mask once a week, when your skin needs a deeper cleanse or an extra hit of moisture. Clay masks are great for drawing out impurities, cream masks help to plump up skin, and sheet masks, which come as pre-soaked cloths, are good for an anti-ageing serum hit.

9. EYE MAKEUP REMOVER

Invest in a specialist eye makeup remover for this delicate area where product is harder to shift. Oil formulas are great for waterproof mascara, but be sure to remove excess oils afterwards. Sensitive eyes and contact lens-wearers should go for water-based removers.

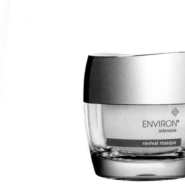
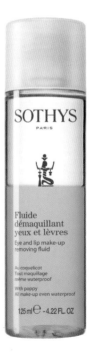

6. Elemis Pro-Collagen Marine Cream

7. Guinot Perfect Radiance Exfoliating Cream

8. Environ Revival Masque

9. Sothys Eye Makeup Removing Fluid

Face charts

Face charts are a fantastic way to play with colour and you can use them at home to plan looks for different occasions without having to wash your face in between every idea you try! They are also great for keeping a record of the looks you have created, as they allow you to note down the products and colours used on each area of the face.

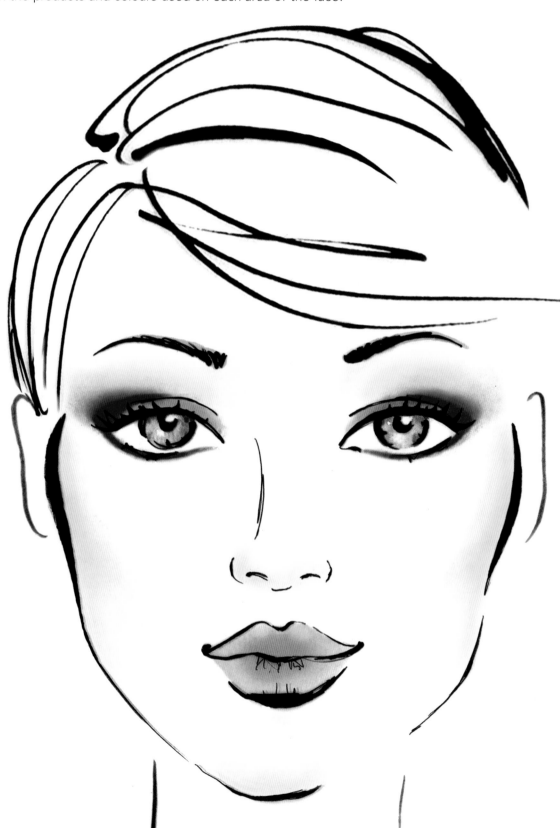

Skin
Honey loose powder,
Soft Dawn bronzer,
Rose Glow blush

Eyes
Orchid cream
eyeshadow, *Cobalt*
loose powder,
Jet gel liner,
Lash Lover mascara

Lips
Starlight lipstick,
Soft Lace lip liner

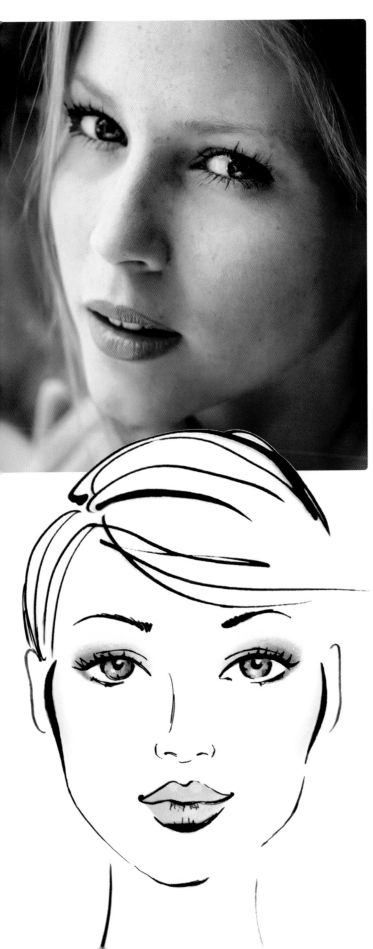

PLANNING A LOOK

Before using real makeup, practise on your chart with coloured pencil. Avoid using liquid or cream makeup, which will smudge. Makeup can be difficult to blend on normal paper; if you want to work like a true pro, use textured watercolour paper, available from art shops.

CREATING YOUR FACE CHART

Trace or photocopy the chart on page 12 or find a blank face chart online to print out. Always tape the paper to a board or table so it doesn't crease or smudge. Some makeup artists like to prime the face chart with loose powder before starting, so that the colours blend more easily. This also helps to create a base colour more like your own skin tone. Use a circular motion to push powders into the paper so they don't smudge. Keep a large, clean, soft brush handy to sweep away any excess powder as you work. With a flat foundation or eyeshadow brush, apply bronzer to create contours around the cheeks, nose, chin and browbone, then add blusher using the same technique.

ADDING COLOUR AND DEFINITION

Next work on the eyes: colour the irises to match your own, then choose shadows to suit your colouring. Using flat brushes, apply the shadows, blending and emphasizing the socket line to create depth. You may find it easier to use smaller, stiffer brushes than you would normally use on your face.

For eyeliner, apply minimal pencil direct to the paper, then use a liner brush to smudge it. To create the lashes, try liquid liner on a very fine brush or just use a black pencil. You don't need to apply mascara – just give an idea of lashes. It's tricky to get brows right with a brow pencil, so use a coloured pencil to create a shape then fill with powder on a liner brush.

Use a flat brush to apply the lipstick. With a liner, add depth around the edges and between the lips. Clear nail polish is great for adding the appearance of gloss on the lips.

When you've finished, use a normal pencil eraser to remove any smudges from around the face. You can then apply a light mist of hairspray to set your look.

Bases

1. PRIMER

Primer cream or liquid preps skin for foundation, smoothing, minimizing lines and pores and helping the base last longer. Look out for oil-control formulas to keep shine at bay and illuminating primers to give dry skin a boost.

2. CONCEALER

Liquid and cream concealers are good for evening-out colour. Blend out the edges of your concealer well with a flat brush. Choose an illuminating formula for undereye circles and try a matt pencil or stick on blemishes.

3. FOUNDATION

Choose a foundation the exact tone of your skin and match the liquid, powder or cream texture to your skin type. Look out for formulas with SPF for daily sun protection. See pages 28–9 for guidance on choosing the right colour and formula for you.

4. BB CREAM / TINTED MOISTURIZER

Lighter than foundation, BB stands for blemish balm and is designed to diffuse imperfections without that full-coverage effect. Great when you're pressed for time, BB creams and tinted moisturizers can be applied and blended with fingers.

5. CORRECTOR / CC CREAM

Colour correctors use opposite tones to neutralize areas of high colour – for example, green correctors on areas of redness, peach tones on pigmentation, and so on. Many brands use the term CC cream to refer to hydrating foundations that give slightly heavier coverage than BB creams, and even out skin tone.

6. TRANSLUCENT POWDER

Fantastic for setting makeup to make it last longer, translucent powder has an invisible finish, reduces shine and minimizes the appearance of imperfections. Dust on with a large powder brush.

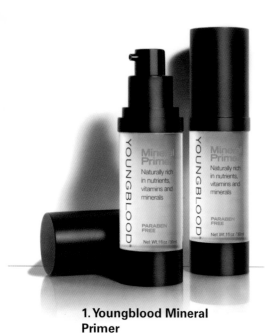

1. Youngblood Mineral Primer

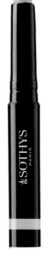

2. Sothys Concealer Pencil

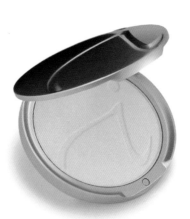

3. Jane Iredale Pure Pressed Base in Golden Glow

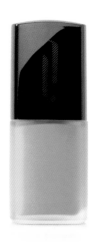

3. Make Up by HD Brows Fluid Foundation in Mink

7. POWDER BRUSH

Far better for applying loose and pressed powders than the puff applicators that come with the products. Dip in powder, tap off excess, then swirl onto the face.

8. BLENDING BRUSH

Good for a full-coverage foundation look. This brush picks up product and lets you work it into the skin for a streak-free, airbrushed effect; also good for cream blush.

9. CONCEALER BRUSH

A slim, tapered or flat brush used for applying concealer and blending out. Domed versions can double as a lip brush.

10. FOUNDATION BRUSH

This brush has a soft, rounded end, great for buffing liquid and cream formulas into the skin in a circular motion, and for blending.

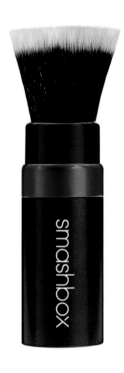

7. Smashbox Telephoto Face Brush

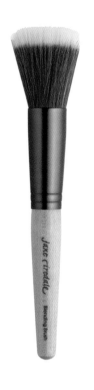

8. Jane Iredale Blending Brush

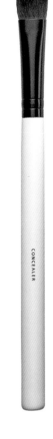

9. Lily Lolo Concealer Brush

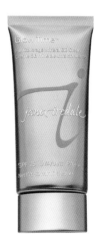

4. Jane Iredale Glow Time Mineral BB Cream

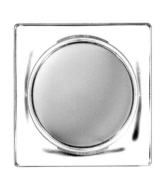

5. Mii Miraculous Colour Corrector in Calm

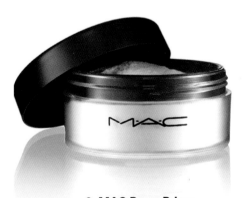

6. MAC Prep+Prime Transparent Finishing Powder

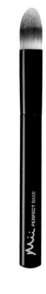

10. Mii Liquid Perfection Base Brush

Definers

1. BRONZER

Pressed powders are most readily found and great for oilier skins, but there are also cream, cream-to-powder, liquid and gel formulas. Apply where the sun would naturally hit the face – the top of the forehead, nose and chin – or use a matt bronzer to shade when contouring.

2. CONTOURING SHADER

Choose a liquid foundation two shades darker than your natural tone and blend over your base below the cheekbones, around the hairline and on either side of the nose and jaw. Or choose a powder formulation – grey undertones help create more shadow – but avoid shimmer. There are some great contouring duo palettes on the market now.

3. HIGHLIGHTER

Choose powder, liquid or cream and use after shading to emphasize the high point of the face, including the cheekbones, Cupid's bow and under the brow. With powder, use a small, fluffy brush, such as an eyeshadow brush, to avoid over-highlighting. White, pearlescent products are good on the palest skins but look very harsh on darker skins, so use peach or gold tones on the latter.

4. CREAM BLUSH

Easier to blend than powder and great for a natural, dewy look, cream blush suits drier or older skins. Apply with fingers, a sponge or a blending brush.

5. POWDER BLUSH

Good for oily or combination skins, powder blush can be built up gradually with a blusher brush. Try plum shades on black skin, peach on mid-tones and sugar pink on pale skin.

6. BLUSHER/BRONZER BRUSH

A soft, long-bristled brush with a rounded end to dust on powder without disturbing foundation.

7. ANGLED BRUSH

Good for contouring or applying blush more precisely, the angle helps to give a controlled diagonal line.

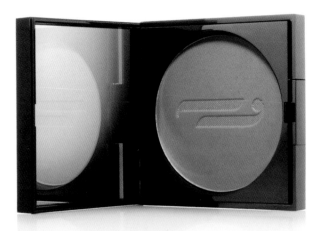

1. Make Up by HD Brows Bronzer in Medium Dark

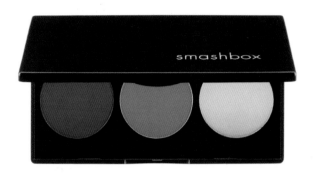

2. Smashbox Step-by-Step Contour Kit

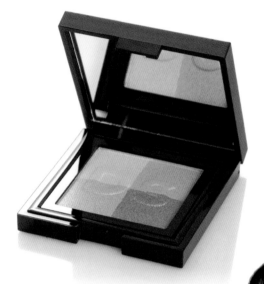

3. Daniel Sandler Radiant Sheen Illuminator

3. Bare Minerals Well Rested Face and Eye Brightener

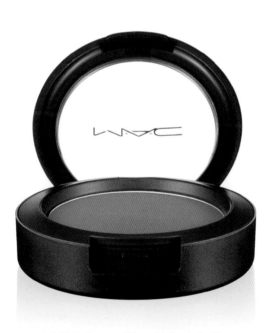

4. MAC Creme Blend Blush in Posey

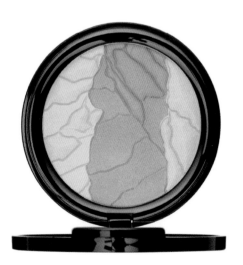

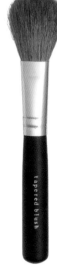

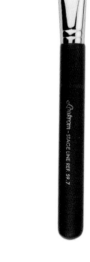

5. Mii Dreamy Duo Cheek Colour in Sweetheart

6. Bare Minerals Tapered Brush

7. Stage Line Professional Laukrom Oblique Blusher Brush

Eyes

1. EYE PRIMER

Just like foundation primer, eye primers create a smooth base. They help eyeshadow stay put for longer (especially loose powder) and stop it from creasing. They can also help bold colours look brighter.

2. PRESSED POWDER SHADOW

Often sold in duos, quads or palettes, pressed powder shadows are your essentials for colouring, highlighting and contouring.

3. CREAM SHADOW

Quicker to blend than powder, these are great for creating solid colour with a sheen. Metallic cream shadows work particularly well. They're also good for layering with powder shadows for lasting, solid colour. They crease easily though, so use sparingly and set with translucent powder.

4. LOOSE POWDER

These give you more product on your brush and create deep colour when gently pressed into a primed lid. They can also be used wet for a foil effect. Metallics are better in loose powder than pressed.

5. PENCIL LINER

Great for smoky eye looks, pencil liners can be smudged and blended then set with powder. Lighter colours can also be blurred to create a subtle, barely-there look.

6. LIQUID LINER

For a fine line or precise flick, nothing beats liquid liners. Use them alone on the upper lid for a vintage winged look or graphic design, or pair an upper-lid flick with pencil liner on the lower lid for a heavier finish.

7. GEL LINER

These bridge the gap between liquid and pencil. They give a deeper colour than pencil with less smudging, but are not as wet as liquid so many people find them easier to apply, using a fine or flat brush.

8. MASCARA

Essential to emphasize the eyes, black mascara suits most people, but go brown if

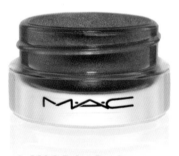

3. MAC Paint Pot in Constructivist

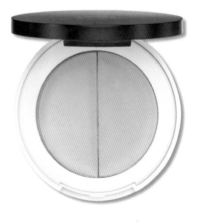

1. Lily Lolo Eye Primer

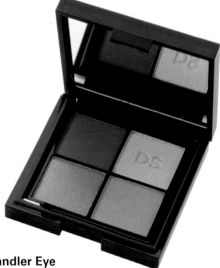

2. Daniel Sandler Eye Shadow Palette in Beyond Sunset

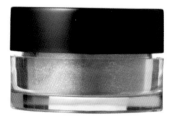

4. Mii Mineral Exquisite Eye Colour in Marvel

you prefer a natural look. Get right to the roots of the lashes, then pull the brush towards the tips with a zig-zag motion, while rolling it inwards to catch every hair. For even fuller lashes, look out for fibre extension mascaras.

9. EYESHADOW BRUSH

Use a small, rounded eyeshadow brush to pick up powder colour, then gently press it on. These brushes are also great for blending shadows.

10. FLAT DEFINER BRUSH

This firmer brush is good for achieving sharper lines with wet or dry powder. It's also great for contouring around the crease of the lid or applying gel liners, if angled. It can double up as a brow brush.

11. EYELINER BRUSH

A thin eyeliner brush can be used to apply gel liners or to turn shadows into liners when applied wet.

12. EYELASH CURLERS

A must for opening up the eye. Use scissor-design versions before applying mascara, or it will clump. Heated lash curlers can often be used after mascara, but they give a less defined finish.

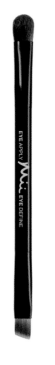

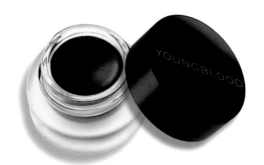

7. Youngblood Incredible Wear Gel Liner in Espresso

9. Mii Eye Define

10. Jane Iredale Angle Definer Brush

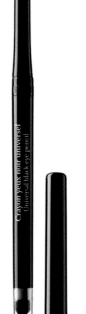

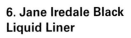

5. Sothys Universal Black Eye Pencil

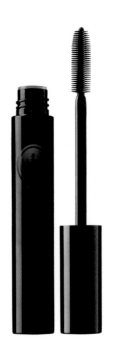

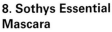

6. Jane Iredale Black Liquid Liner

8. Sothys Essential Mascara

11. Make Up by HD Brows Eyeliner Brush

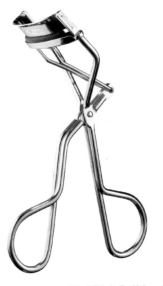

12. MAC Full Lash Curler

Lips

1. LIP SCRUB

For a smooth start, use a sugary scrub once a week to slough off dry skin – or make your own by adding a little sugar to your favourite lip balm.

2. LIP PRIMER

A base to hydrate and create a smooth canvas that helps lipstick stay put. Also helps to stop colour bleeding or feathering on older lips.

3. LIP LINER

This pencil can be used before lipstick or after, to crisp the outline. Invest in a good sharpener to keep lines precise. Blend out for a softer finish.

4. LIP GLOSS

The quickest way to add colour to lips; use on days when time is tight or apply over lipstick in the centre of the lips to give the illusion of fullness.

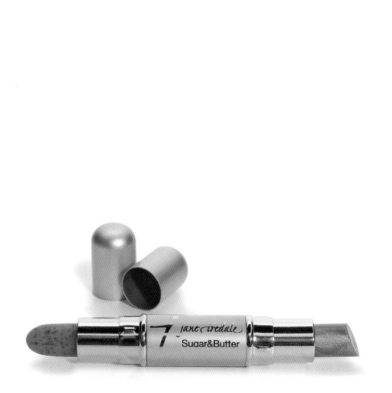

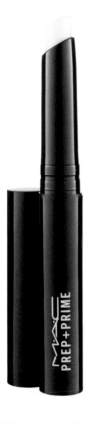

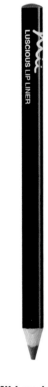

1. Jane Iredale Sugar & Butter

2. MAC Prep & Prime

3. Mii Luscious Lip Liner

5. LIPSTICK

Choose a shade to suit your skin tone (see pages 68–9) and apply with a lip brush. Cream formulas give stronger colour. Sheer colours are great for a more natural look and for adding volume. Try lip crayons if you want a product that's faster to apply, but has a less precise finish.

6. LIP AND CHEEK STAIN

Excellent multi-tasking products, cheek and lip stains can double up as lipstick, blush and even eyeshadow when space and time are tight. Some lip stains come in a felt tip-style container – for use on lips only. These work well as a base and help to avoid patchy colour as your lipstick wears off.

7. LIP BRUSH

This small, flat brush with a rounded tip can be used to apply lipstick with a more even coverage than you get straight from the bullet. Start in the centre of the lips and buff outwards.

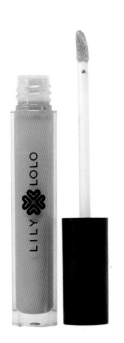

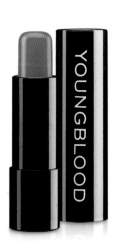

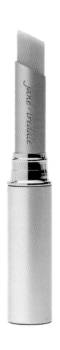

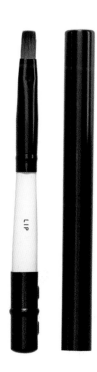

4. Lily Lolo Scandalips Natural Lip Gloss in English Rose

5. Youngblood Hydrating Lip Crème

6. Jane Iredale Forever Pink Just Kissed Lip and Cheek Stain

7. Lily Lolo Lip Brush

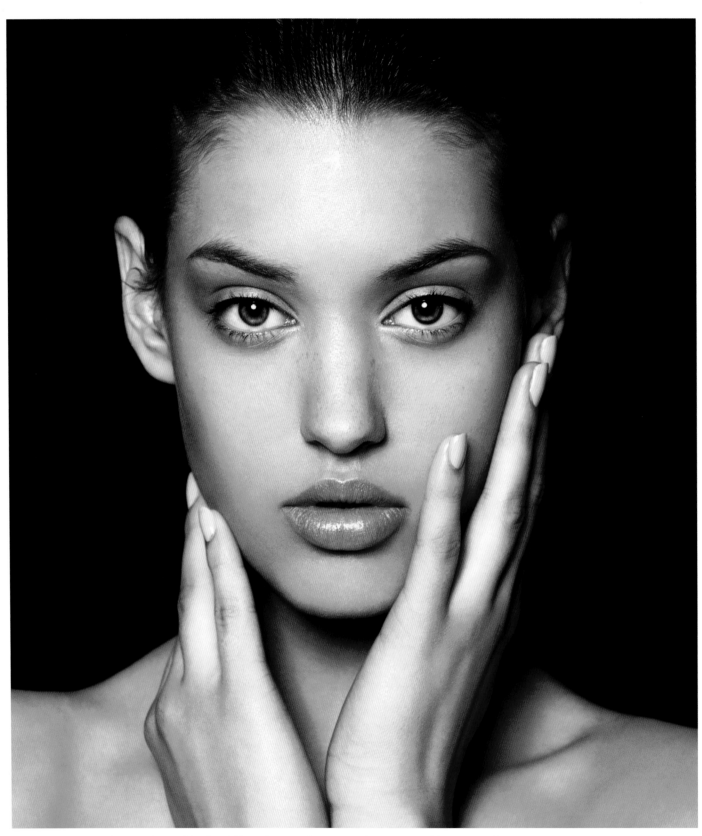

Flawless skin is the product of luck, skill and, most importantly, a great skincare regime

Chapter Two

Flawless Base

If you've seen any of those 'celebs before they were airbrushed' photos you will know that not even Beyoncé wakes up with picture-perfect, flawless skin. If Photoshop isn't an option, there are plenty of professional cheats to help you achieve an even base.

A flawless base has to start with skincare. If you layer foundation on skin that is too oily, it will just slide off. Cake it onto dry skin and you'll be left with a flaky mess. But if you exfoliate regularly, cleanse well and keep moisturizer light before applying your base, you'll be off to a good start. If you're still having problems achieving that natural-looking glow, try using a corrector. Green-based concealers or colour correctors are great for toning down redness around the nose and cheeks, while rose and coral tones can help correct dark circles. Yellow can cover purplish tones in the skin, while lilac will brighten sallow, yellowish complexions.

Flawless base is all about layering, but the beauty of it is you can choose the layers you need. For full coverage that will last all day, you might layer concealer, primer, foundation and powder, while for young skins with fewer problem zones, a touch of well-blended concealer may be enough on its own. Or, in that minute before you dash out of the door to work, you can cheat an even skin with a BB cream.

Like any makeup look, the concept of perfect skin changes according to trends; makeup artists might be asked to create an even-toned matt finish one season and a dewy, fresh-faced look the next. Clever contouring with shadow and highlighter has produced some of the strongest looks in recent years; similarly, illuminated skin that appears to glow from within is in high demand. All these looks can be achieved at home, with a few insider tips from the professionals.

Skin prep

Creating beautiful, flawless skin is about so much more than concealer and foundation. If you don't have a smooth, hydrated base to work from, your makeup can look patchy and won't last the day. A regular skincare routine paired with good nutrition is the only way to change the skin long term, as this will work on the deeper layers. But there are still some quick-fix ways to use skincare to prep the face for a smooth finish.

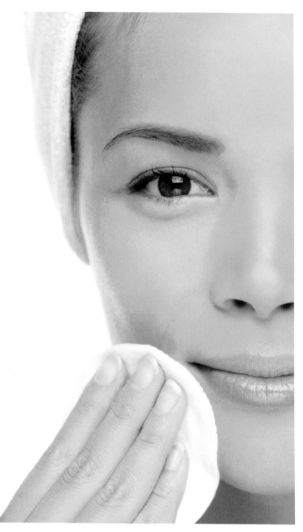

JO COLETTA'S PRE-SHOOT ROUTINE

Prep

Cleanse In case the model's skin reacts, I always thoroughly cleanse twice with a non-alcohol cleanser. I love Bioderma's Sensibio and Cosmetics à La Carte Total Lift Off. I soak soft cotton pads with the cleanser and wipe over the face, neck and ears.

Tone Spritz toner directly onto the face, then absorb excess with cotton pads. I only ever use Dermalogica Multi-Active Toner.

Serum I always use a serum after toning. Kiehl's do great ones for lifting, pore tightening and reducing fine lines. This is when I really start to work the product into the skin to create a flawless base. I use a stippling makeup brush to do this.

Moisturize Choose a moisturizer to suit your skin type, but stick to a light formulation if applying it just before your makeup. I use a stippling brush for this too and spend a good few minutes applying the serum and moisturizer. Adding the product to the end of the brush and applying to the skin in small soft circular movements really works the product into the skin and is like a mini-massage.

PROFILE
JO COLETTA

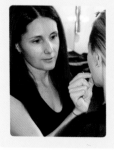

Jo Coletta is a freelance hair and makeup artist whose work credits include regular online and print editorials, advertising campaigns, as well as doing makeup for TV shows and celebrities. She specializes in makeup for men, with a strong focus on skincare.

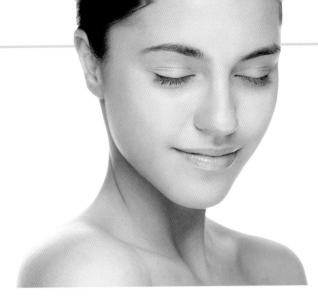

Lips Use a sugar lip scrub and really work it in with your finger. Remove it with cleanser then apply a lip balm quite heavily and leave it to soak into the lips. Blot with a tissue before applying your lip makeup. This is a great lip prep, especially before applying a matt lipstick, as it removes all dead skin and makes the lips really smooth.

Correct

After cleansing, toning and moisturizing, I assess the model's skin. Instead of just covering with a heavy foundation or concealer, I try to correct any problems such as redness, acne, dark circles or open pores.

Redness I use products with a yellow or green tint, such as Clinique Super City Block or Dermalogica Redness Relief, to neutralize the colour. Don't use a product that is too green as it can make the skin quite ashen. Apply it only to the area where needed and blend with a soft blending brush. Areas where this is often needed are the forehead, around the nose and nostrils, the centre of your chin under your bottom lip and on broken capillaries. For photographic work, I also use it to neutralize redness on the ears and hands.

Uneven skin I love smoothing primers such as Giorgio Armani Fluid Master Primer to even out the skin tone. Start in the centre of the face and work your way outwards using the fingertips or a blending sponge.

Visible pores Try a smoothing primer balm such as Benefit Pore-fessional.

Puffiness If the undereyes look puffy and tired, apply cooling undereye pads. My faves are by Skyn Iceland.

Undereye dark circles Use a peach, pink or orange corrector before applying concealer, working the product into the skin and then blending.

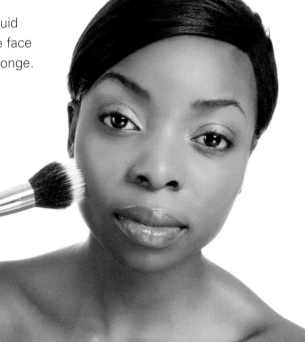

Concealing

Concealer can be used to cover dark circles, redness, spots, pigmentation or any areas of the face where you'd just like to even out the tone. Most MUAs use concealer underneath foundation, but you can always add another layer on top of your base for extra coverage on problem zones such as pimples, as long as it's blended well.

Before concealing, prep your face to get rid of any dryness or excess oil. Wash with a gentle cleanser, then tone and moisturize so that your concealer will go on smoothly. Use a very light eye cream under your eyes.

The type of concealer you use should vary depending on the area you want to even out. For high-colour zones, such as redness around the nose, use a liquid concealer that's the same shade or one shade lighter than your skin tone. Apply it using a concealer brush or your finger, dotting it around the crease of the nose. Then blend it using a flat brush. Use your fingers at the very edges to blend in the last bits. Always tap, rather than rub when blending to avoid rubbing the concealer off. Set it with a light, yellow-based powder. Use a powder that's a shade lighter than your usual face powder as it will darken when it meets the wet concealer.

For areas of dark pigmentation, a cream concealer will give stronger coverage. Dot it carefully onto the pigmented area, and blend.

To cover dark circles under the eyes, specialist undereye concealers work best as they contain illuminators which counteract shadowing and brighten the area. Some also have a corrective pink or peach tone that will help to neutralize the purple and grey shadows. Alternatively, you can use a separate corrector first then follow with liquid concealer before setting with light powder.

For pimples, pencil concealers really come into their own as you can apply them precisely and get great coverage. If the area is very red, try neutralizing first with a green corrector.

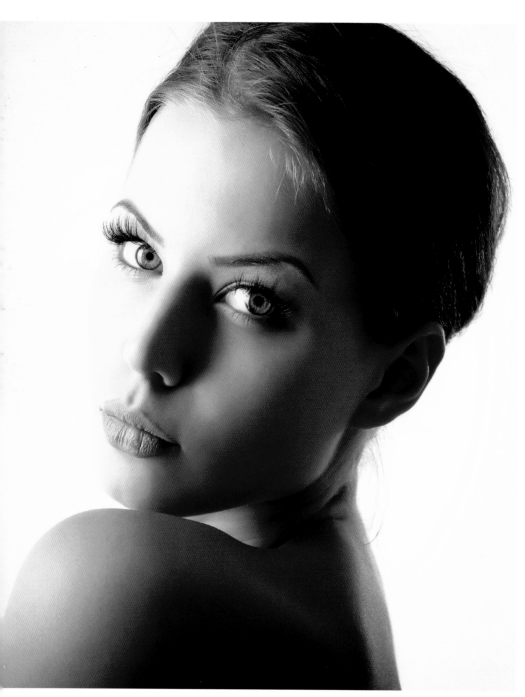

JEN HUNTER'S TOP TIPS FOR CONCEALING

1. When correcting dark circles under the eyes, use a salmon-coloured corrector if you have olive or yellow-toned skin and a rose shade for paler tones. This will leave a neutral tone to conceal.

2. Use your ring finger to dab on concealer. This will leave a natural coverage that won't feel too heavy on the skin.

3. If you want to cover blemishes on your face, use a concealer the same colour as your foundation rather than a lighter one, so that it looks as natural as possible.

4. For redness around the nose or on the cheeks, try a green-based concealer; this will correct the redness before you apply foundation.

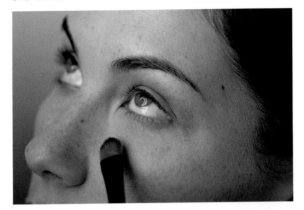

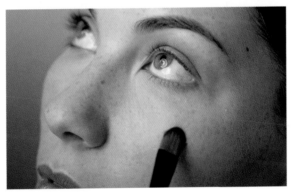

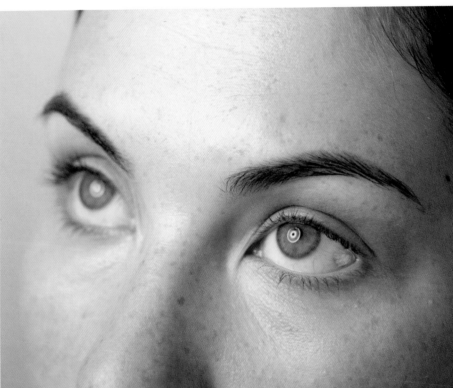

Jen Hunter demos undereye concealing with liquid concealer

PROFILE
JEN HUNTER

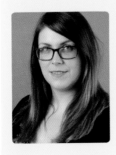

Jen Hunter is a professional makeup artist who provides makeup services ranging from bridal to beauty, and from special effects to personal makeup lessons. Her talents saw her win the Professional Beauty Makeup Specialist of the Year Award in 2014.

Pro's tip

If your skin is prone to dehydration and your concealer looks cakey when it dries, try mixing it with a little foundation to thin it before applying.

Choosing foundation

With cream, liquid, mousse, pressed and loose powder and even cream/powder foundations on the shelves in every shade imaginable, picking the perfect colour and formulation of foundation for your skin can be daunting.

Remember, the best foundation will disappear on your face – the shade will blend seamlessly and the formula will melt in without greasiness or chalkiness. While it's fine to go cheap on fashion colours such as eyeshadow, foundation is the one product it's worth splashing out on, so take your time testing. If you're not sure about shades, ask the advice of a professional at the makeup counter or in your local salon. She will be able to analyse the tones and textures of your skin, with no obligation to buy.

CHOOSING COLOURS

To test colours before buying, always go barefaced to the store so you're matching your skin and not your makeup.

THE TONE

Choose colours to test based on the underlying tone of your skin as well as how light or dark it appears. Skin is made up of lots of different tones, but most people can determine a dominant undertone. A good way to check whether yours is warm or cool is to look at the inside of your wrist. On cool tones, the veins will appear blue whereas they will have a greenish hue through warmer skins. If your skin is cool, look for pink or blue-based foundations; if it is warm, start with more yellow-based shades. Remember, the colour of your skin does not determine the underlying tone. While cool tones are usually associated with pale skin and warm with darker skin, many black and Asian skins also have a cool undertone, and vice versa.

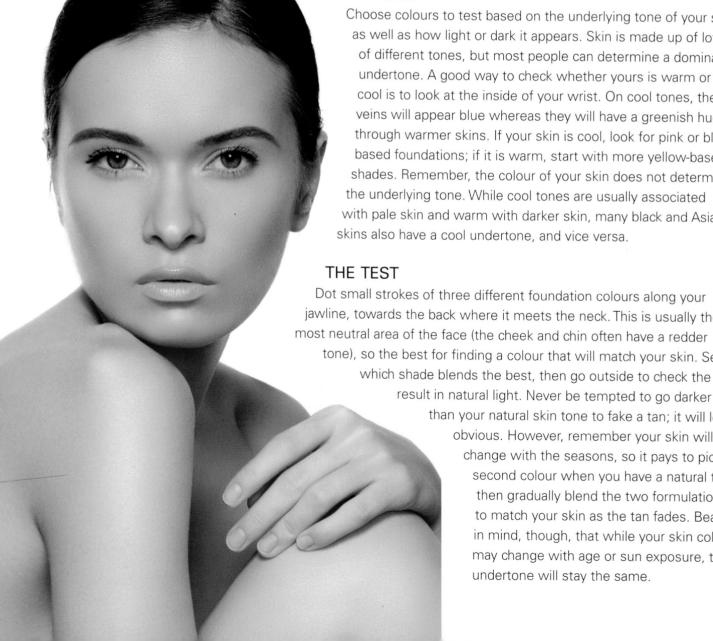

THE TEST

Dot small strokes of three different foundation colours along your jawline, towards the back where it meets the neck. This is usually the most neutral area of the face (the cheek and chin often have a redder tone), so the best for finding a colour that will match your skin. See which shade blends the best, then go outside to check the result in natural light. Never be tempted to go darker than your natural skin tone to fake a tan; it will look obvious. However, remember your skin will change with the seasons, so it pays to pick a second colour when you have a natural tan, then gradually blend the two formulations to match your skin as the tan fades. Bear in mind, though, that while your skin colour may change with age or sun exposure, the undertone will stay the same.

FORMULATIONS

Your usual skin condition should determine the formula you go for. Foundation can balance skin's texture as well as its colour, so look for formulations that counteract your skin concerns to get that flawless finish. Your skin condition can change with age, often becoming drier as you get older. The environment may also have an effect. Cold winters can mean dry, flaky patches, while warm summers can make skin oilier and more prone to breakouts, so you may need to switch your foundation as the seasons change.

OILY SKIN

Look for mattifying formulas. Seek out water-based (rather than oil-based) liquids and creams or try a mousse formula. These give a lighter coverage and dry fast with a matt finish. Loose powder is great for light coverage, but make sure your skin is cleansed and oil-free before applying so that it doesn't cake. Carry blotting sheets in your handbag to absorb excess oil during the day without having to layer on more product.

DRY SKIN

For a light finish go for the extra hydration of a tinted moisturizer or BB cream. For a fuller coverage, liquid foundations with a hydrating formula are your best bet. Steer clear of powders as they will make your skin look flaky or chalky.

COMBINATION SKIN

If you have an oily T-zone, but are prone to dryness elsewhere, look for equalizing formulas. Try a liquid or cream with both hydrating and anti-shine claims. Smart formulas contain ingredients that work only where they are needed, absorbing excess oil on your forehead and chin while hydrating your cheeks. A light dusting of a mineral loose powder over shiny areas will absorb excess oil without blocking pores or irritating the skin.

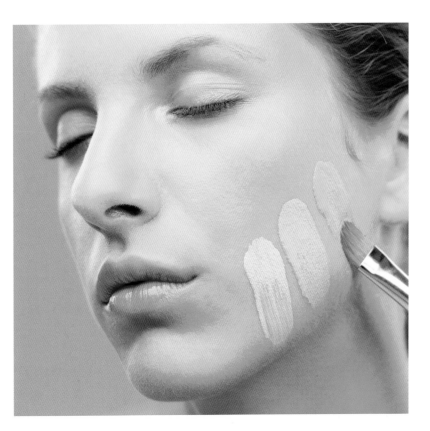

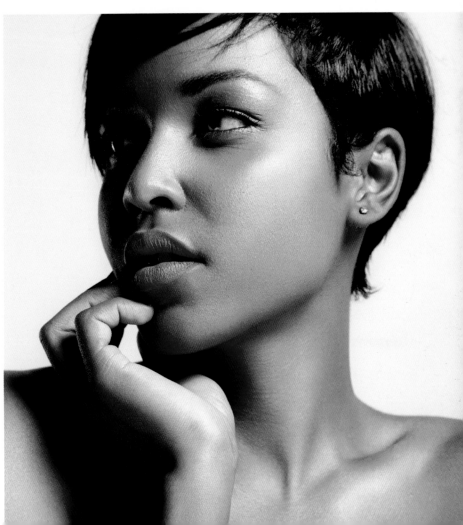

Applying primer and foundation

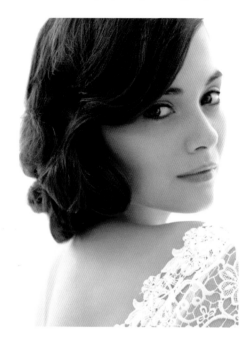

For a flawless finish, primer is essential. Not only does it create a base for your foundation to ensure that your makeup lasts longer, it can also smooth the complexion by filling in any imperfections such as open pores and fine lines. If you have dry skin, choose a primer with anti-ageing ingredients as this will keep skin moisturized throughout the day. For oilier skin, choose primers that are oil-free and mattifying to keep shine under control.

Match your chosen primer with the right foundation: oily skins suit a more matt liquid or powder-finish foundation, whereas a liquid formulation with light-reflective properties is best for more mature or drier skin types. Normal skin types can choose either, depending on the finish they prefer.

According to pro makeup artist Sarah Brock, the best tools for applying these products are a foundation brush and your fingers. 'I don't like sponges, as they soak up too much product and tend to rub the product away rather than blend it onto the skin,' she says.

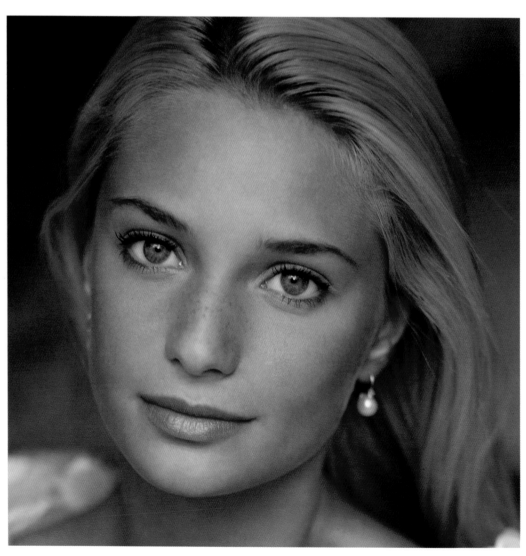

Flawless, natural-looking skin created with primer and foundation by Sarah Brock

SARAH BROCK'S TOP TIPS FOR FLAWLESS PRIMER AND FOUNDATION

1. Apply your primer after your moisturizer. Avoid greasy moisturizers, as they will stop the primer going on evenly. For best results, smooth primer over your face in a thin, even layer, using your fingers.

2. Using a brush, apply foundation to the centre of the face and blend outwards. Take your time doing this; it's essential to cover all areas of your face, including the eyelids.

3. Remember, foundation is meant to even out your skin tone, not cover imperfections and blemishes. Using your brush, apply it in a thin layer all over your face, then blend well using your fingers.

4. Less is more: apply both products in thin, even layers, as it is easier to add more product than to take it away. Thin layers will give a more natural, dewy finish to your skin.

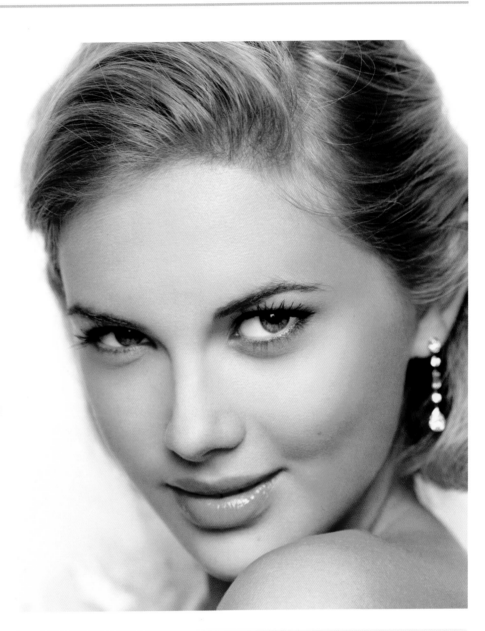

PROFILE
SARAH BROCK

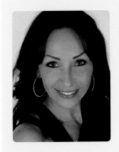

Sarah Brock is a leading bridal makeup artist. She has been selected by top beauty editors, journalists and celebrities to do the makeup on their wedding days and has collaborated with the biggest names in bridal fashion ad campaigns. She has created makeup looks for 22 covers of Condé Nast *Brides* magazine, as well as numerous fashion and makeover shoots.

Illuminating the skin

Have you ever watched celebrities on the red carpet and wondered how they get their skin to look so radiant, as though it's lit from within? To create glowing, luminescent skin you need to prepare a flawless base and keep the layering light and fresh.

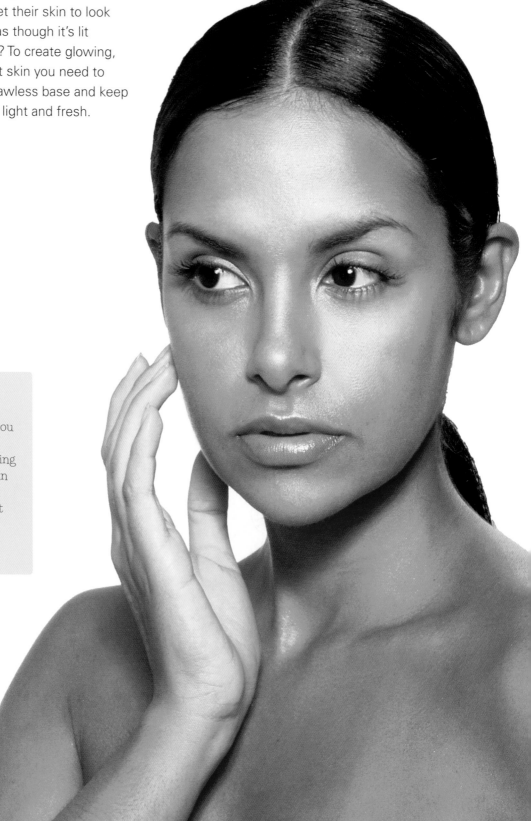

Pro's tip

If you have oily skin, you can stabilize it by first applying some mattifying primer to the nose, chin and forehead. This will ensure the look doesn't slip from glowing to greasy during the day.

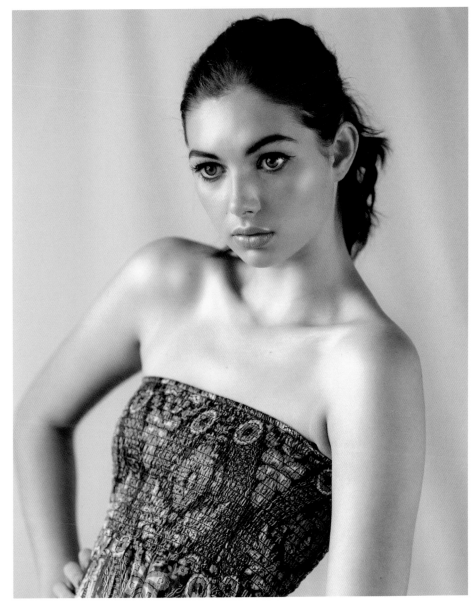

Glowing skin by Catherine Bailey

CATHERINE BAILEY'S STEP-BY-STEP GUIDE TO GLOWING SKIN

1. Start with a smoothing primer such as Clarins Instant Smooth Perfecting Touch where needed, to ensure the surface of your skin is totally even, as the light-reflective products you'll use to create this look tend to highlight flaws such as fine lines and open pores.

2. Apply a very light layer of a sheer foundation which allows your natural skin tone to show through, and conceal only where needed. I like Chanel Vitalumière Acqua because it's ultra-light and gives a really fresh finish.

3. Dot a natural-toned cream or liquid blusher onto the apples of your cheeks and blend thoroughly, so that your skin looks like it's glowing from within.

4. Smooth a pearly but not frosty highlighting liquid onto the middle of your forehead, down the bridge of your nose and across the tops of your cheekbones, and blend well. On this model, I used Becca Shimmering Skin Perfector in Moonstone.

5. Set your base with a sheer dusting of a light-reflecting powder such as Hourglass Ambient Lighting Powder.

PROFILE
CATHERINE BAILEY

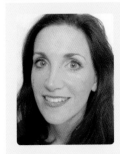

Catherine Bailey has done the makeup for numerous fashion shoots, and her work has been featured in top bridal magazines and blogs.

Contouring with foundation

Clever contouring can bring out your best features, making your face look slimmer and your features more chiselled. Shadowing will give the illusion of hollowing out your cheekbones, but contouring should always be subtle, so stick to matt shades and avoid orangey bronzers.

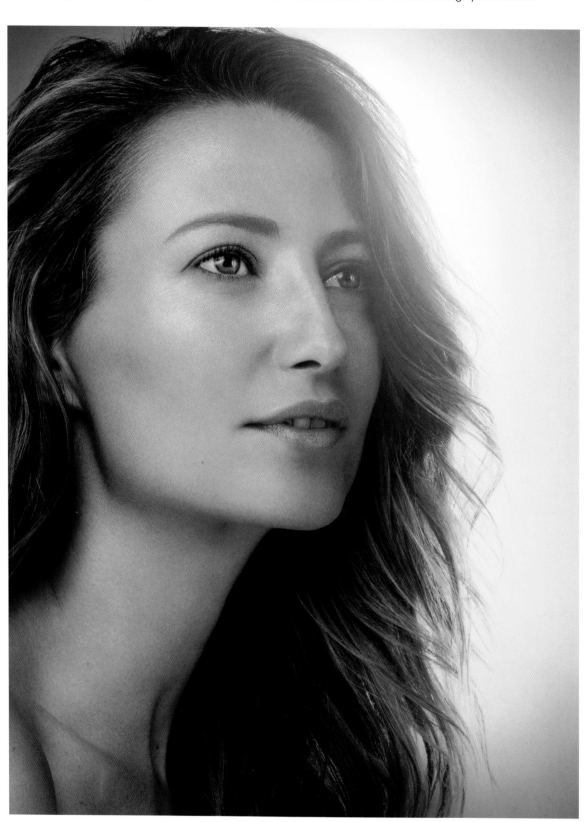

Subtle foundation contouring by Sarah Jane Froom using Bare Minerals

SARAH JANE FROOM'S STEP-BY-STEP GUIDE TO CONTOURING

1. Apply a very fine layer of your normal shade of foundation.

2. Feel for the contours of your face and apply a darker shade of foundation directly underneath your cheekbone, extending from the centre of your ear in a slightly downward motion. Use a brush for greater control.

3. Use a small eyeshadow brush to softly line both sides of your nose with the darker shade of foundation. If you have a long nose, apply a little more under the tip to shorten the appearance.

4. Feel your jaw then use your brush to apply your contour colour below the jawbone. Make sure you don't apply any colour to the actual bone. However, if your jaw is large, you can bring the contour colour up on either side of the chin to make it appear less bold.

5. To slim the appearance of your face, blend contour colour into your hairline. Use your fingers as well as the brush to make sure the colour is well blended and you can't see any product.

6. To give the look even more impact, use a highlighter pen down the centre of the nose, the centre of the forehead, under the eyes, at the top of the cheeks, the centre of the chin, the browbone, above the lip and on the lower eyelids.

7. Using your fingers, gently press and roll, then buff and blend using clean brushes so that the dark and light merge and you see no harsh lines.

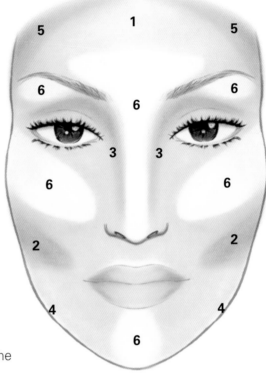

A contouring face chart by Bare Minerals

PROFILE
SARAH JANE FROOM

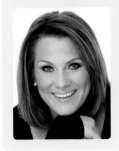

Sarah Jane Froom has worked on editorial shoots for top glossy magazines including *Tatler*, *Vogue* and *Hello*, and with designers such as Vivienne Westwood and Chanel. Since 2006 she has been the international makeup artist for Bare Minerals, travelling the world with the brand.

Pro's tip

Pearly highlighters look great on pale skins, but medium and dark complexions need a warmer golden tone. This creates a natural glow and avoids looking washed out.

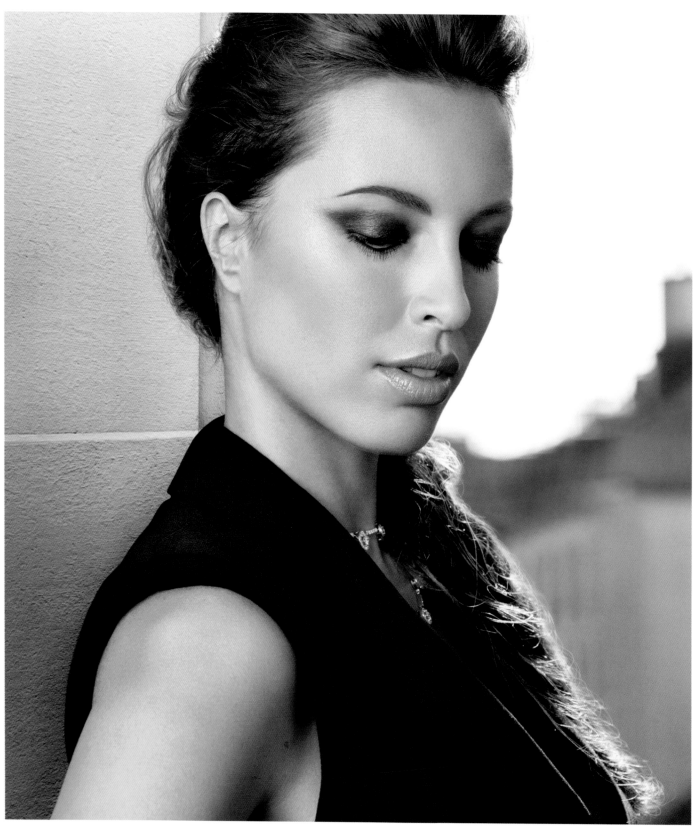

A standout smoky eye and defined brow applied over a softly contoured base by Sothys

Chapter Three

Eye Time

If you want your makeup to make a statement, remember – it's all in the eyes. From the classic smoky effect to bold, bright colours, strong detail can make your eyes look bigger and lift your whole face. But don't go bold without mastering the basics and incorporating some professional cheats. Take the time to play with eye primers and with layering cream and powder shadows for long-lasting looks. Choose shades that complement your eye colour for a subtle smoulder, or clash colours to really draw attention to your eyes.

Ever since Cleopatra got busy with the charcoal in Ancient Egypt, women have been embellishing their eyes, using shading, highlighting and elongated lines to create or emphasize shape. From the rounded, wide-eyed look of the 1920s to the feline, almond shape of the 1950s, shadow and liner have set the look of the time.

New trends bring with them new tools, such as enriched brow pencils and precision application graphic liners, while new formulations offer a lasting finish that will help to keep that carefully blended smoky eye makeup in place all night long.

Choosing eyeshadows

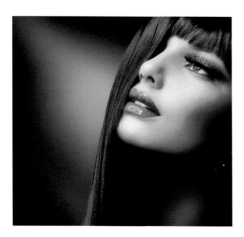

Don't be tempted to choose an eyeshadow just because it's on-trend or one of your favourite colours or textures. If it doesn't suit your skin tone and eye colour, it can work against them. Choosing the right eyeshadow can make the difference between a bright, healthy-looking skin tone and a dull, lifeless complexion.

Your skin tone can be just as important as your eye colour when choosing eye products. Colours that provide a subtle contrast to your eye colour will work well, as long as they are not too light or dark for your skin tone. In general, warm shadows suit cool eye colours and vice versa; but, if you want to play it safe, you can't go far wrong with soft neutrals as they suit almost any eye colour and skin tone.

MELANIE DOYLE'S TOP TIPS TO CHOOSING EYE COLOURS

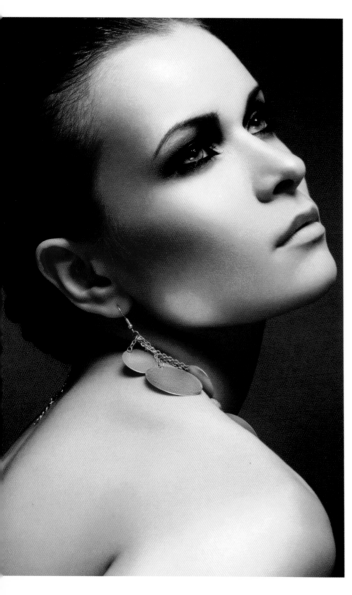

Brown eyes

Brown eyes suit most shades, especially soft neutrals. Cool colours, such as blues and greens, enhance warm brown eyes. Try mixing a little blue and green together for a dramatic effect. Metallic textures and glitters are perfect as they lift the darkness of brown eyes without being too dramatic.

Green eyes

Golden brown, taupe, rich purple, peach and violet shades will set off green eyes and emphasize them as a striking feature. Purples work best of all, but don't use too many shades of purple together or you could end up with a bruised or bloodshot look! Remember, sometimes less is more.

Blue eyes

Try warm shades of brown, taupe, gold, plum and peach. Blue eyeshadow can dull your natural eye colour, but if you mix it up a little and use gold with a touch of blue, this can work beautifully. Blue eyes can be icy looking, so try cream textured shadows to help warm them. These work best on young eyes, though, as they tend to crease and can age older eyes.

Grey eyes

Choose charcoal, brown and soft purple or violet shades. Warm shades really enhance grey eyes. Use glitter to add a little sparkle and help lift the coloured flecks that you tend to find in grey irises.

Fair skin and blonde hair

Choose: black mascara; black or navy eye pencil; natural, soft eyeshadow colours; light brown brow pencil and shadow.

Pale skin and red hair

Choose: warm, brown eyeliner and mascara colours; eyeshadow products with copper and bronze undertones.

Mid-toned skin and brown hair

Choose: dark, rich colours for eyeshadow such as jewel tones of plum or forest green; liner and mascara in black or chocolate brown.

Olive or mixed-race skin

Choose: warm browns or eyeshadows with chocolate, silver, bronze or olive undertones; black mascara.

Asian skin

Choose: black eyeliner; cool dark grey or silver eyeshadow colours; iridescent and sheer pale textures; black mascara.

Black skin

Choose: shimmer beige, deep brown, copper, bronze and mahogany eyeshadows; metallic textures; inky blue-black mascara.

Mature skin, grey hair

Choose: neutral tones; matt shades; soft brown liners and mascaras. Avoid strong colours and iridescent or glitter textures.

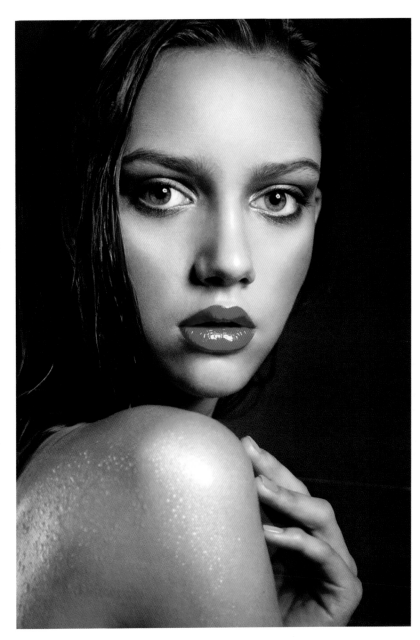

PROFILE
MELANIE DOYLE

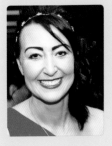

Melanie Doyle is a freelance educator for several makeup brands. She has worked on TV dramas such as *Downton Abbey* and been makeup artist to numerous TV stars and for red carpet events such as the National Television Awards. She is head judge for the NMUAUK professional makeup artist and student competitions.

The smoky eye

A smoky eye can add drama and sophistication to any look. It's a classic, sexy style that suits everyone, but it can be tough to master. The key is to prep well, build colour up gradually and blend like your life depends on it!

For a really dramatic eye you'll use a lot of dark product, so try applying your eye makeup before your foundation. This way, if specks of dark powder fall onto your cheek you can easily wipe them away without taking any base off.

JEN HUNTER'S STEP-BY-STEP GUIDE TO THE SMOKY EYE

1. Start with a clean eyelid and build up your base, beginning with a primer to help your eyeshadow stay on longer. Using a kohl eye pencil, apply it to the outside half of the lid, then use a soft eyeshadow blending brush to work it in.

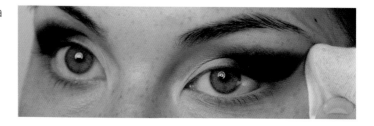

2. Take a grey powder shadow and apply it over the kohl, extending it beyond the edges and blending well. Next apply your lightest eyeshadow powder, taking it right into the inner corners of the eye and up to the edge of the grey, blending the two colours.

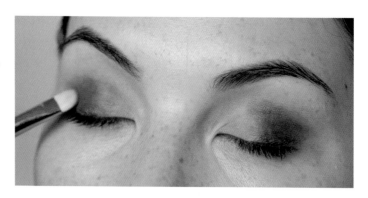

3. Use the brush to place black shadow in the outer corners of the eye, leaving a strip of grey in the centre. Take the black out and up slightly towards the tail of the eyebrow, blending as you go.

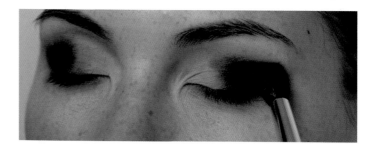

4. Clean up the edges by wrapping a tissue around your finger and using it to dust away excess powder. Add more of your palest shadow above the black and up to the brow bone, to highlight.

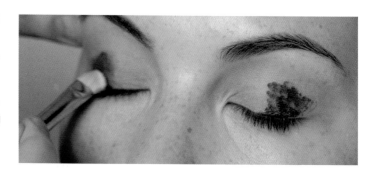

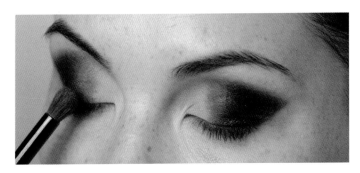

5. Try blending a small amount of dark metallic shadow into the centre of each eyelid to create depth. Using an eyeshadow blending brush in circular motions, make sure that you don't have any harsh lines and your colours blend.

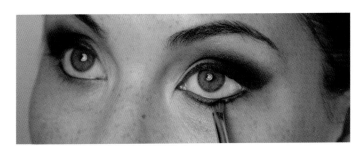

6. Take a kohl liner close to the top lashes and inside the lashline on the bottom lid. Using a fine liner brush with black powder, create a line beneath the bottom lashes and blend.

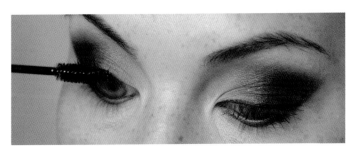

7. Finish with black mascara on the top and bottom lashes.

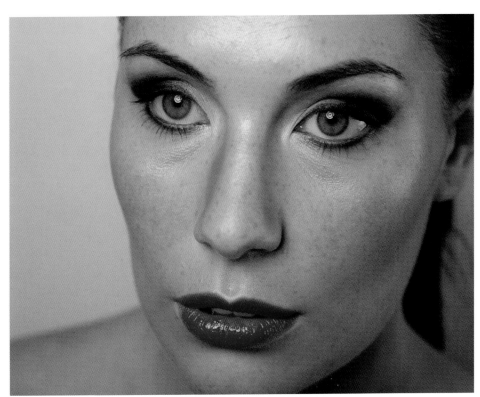

Pro's tip

Remember, it's always easier to start with less eyeshadow and add more than to remove excess when you have finished.

A twist on the smoky eye

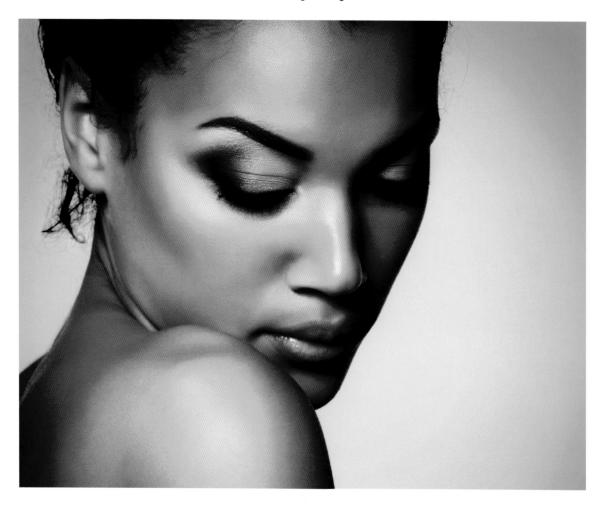

The smoky eye is a timeless favourite, but it can quickly get boring if it becomes your go-to party look. Once you've mastered the classic smoky, you can try softening it for a wearable daytime look by using browns rather than blacks or pumping up the volume with metallics and liquid liner. You can mix it up a little with on-trend seasonal colours so that your makeup changes with your wardrobe and never gets stuck in a rut. Try smoky blues in spring and copper or emerald shades in autumn for a fresh take on the look.

Pro's tip

Try using cream shadow instead of powder for a mess-free smoky eye. Apply pencil liner first, then blend cream shadow into it, working it outwards across the upper lid and below the lower lashline with a blending brush. Then clean up any smudgy edges with a cotton bud.

PROFILE
DANIELLE DRURY

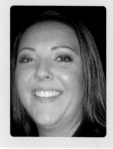

Danielle Drury has been national education manager for Parisian makeup and skincare brand Sothys since 2008. She trains makeup artists and beauty therapists to create new looks with the salon-professional products.

DANIELLE DRURY'S STEP-BY-STEP GUIDE TO AN AUTUMNAL SMOKY EYE

1. Create a flawless base to let your high-impact eye makeup really stand out. Apply foundation with a brush to clean, prepped skin, then correct any areas that need more coverage before applying a dusting of fixing powder using a powder brush. Contour and highlight with powder and add a soft coral blush.

2. Alternatively, apply a light base to the eyes first, using an eyeshadow brush. Next choose a soft matt taupe eyeshadow and apply it to the upper eyelid, taking it down beneath the lower lashline.

3. Then, using the same brush, apply a deep, iridescent emerald shade such as Sothys' Reflet Nocturne to the eye socket and outer corners, working inwards into the socket and onto the eye contour bone. Blend carefully into the taupe.

4. Apply a soft brown eye pencil along the upper and lower lashlines. Blend to create a smoky effect using an eyeshadow brush, then complete your seasonal smoky eye look with a coat of black mascara. Or apply strip lashes for even more impact.

5. Use a mid-brown brow pencil to fill and shape the brows, then blend using an eyebrow brush.

6. As the autumnal smoky eye is softer than a classic black and grey, you can afford to go bolder on the lips. Choose a coppery red to keep it autumnal, and don't be afraid of a shimmer.

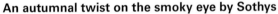

An autumnal twist on the smoky eye by Sothys

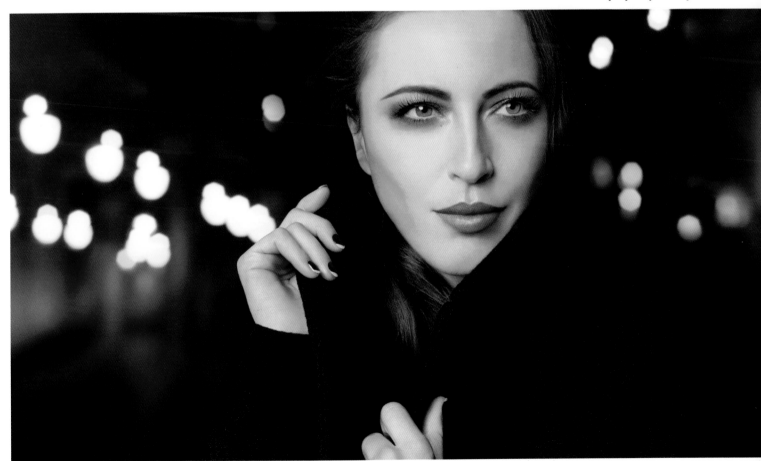

Metallics

For a really high-fashion look, glossy metallic shadows work well either alone for a classy shimmer or with lots of dark liner for a rock look. Warm gold shadows will flatter any skin tone. Silver-based metallics can be harsher on the skin; blondes can carry these off, but brunettes should usually stick to gold-based metallics. For the best effect, you'll need to layer loose powder over a cream shadow to make sure the colour lasts. Match the cream shadow to your skin tone for a light wash of metallic, or use the same colour as the powder shadow for a more heavily pigmented look.

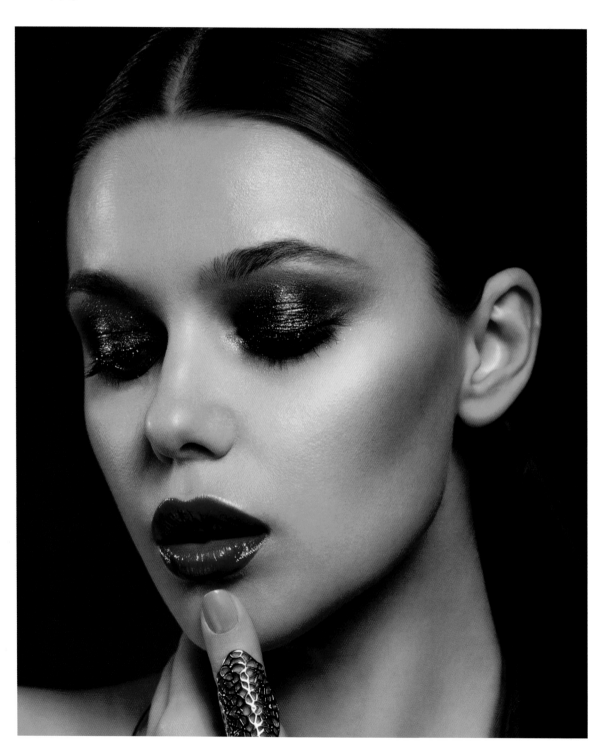

SALINA THIND'S STEP-BY-STEP GUIDE TO PERFECTING THE METALLIC EYE

1. Start with a clean eyelid – don't use concealer or foundation as a base because it adds an oily barrier. You don't want any greasiness; it will make the powder slide and crease.

2. Apply the cream eyeshadow first. Choose one that dries completely rather than a cream that leaves a tacky finish, and look for crease-resistant formulas. Take the colour over the whole lid and into both corners of the eye. For a more dramatic look, add a little under the lower lid too.

3. Then go straight in with the pigment. Use a loose powder shadow and push it carefully into the cream using an eyeshadow brush. I tend to use MAC or Bobbi Brown as they do some great metallics.

4. A liquid liner flick is great to finish off the look, especially if you intend to keep the lips subtle. Line the inside of the lower lid too. Lots of black mascara is good for a really high-impact metallic eye. If you want to go strong on the lips, then metallic shadow and mascara with no liner works best.

5. For a metallic eye, avoid shimmer on the rest of the face, especially the lips – a matt lip works really well to contrast, but you can also get away with a gloss. Nude tones let the eyes dominate the look. Alternatively, pair a gold eye with a bright red lip for a high-fashion look which is great for Christmas. Wine colours work really well too.

6. If you're doing a strong eye and lip together, then stay away from blush, but do a slight contour. Some people are scared of adding anything more to the face when there is strong makeup on the eyes and lips, but if you have a flawless base with no colour it can look very flat. It's worth warming up the face with some soft contouring on the cheeks.

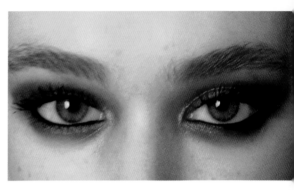

Variations on the metallic eye look, by Salina Thind

Pro's tips

Metallic browns and golds will make blue eyes 'pop'. For brown eyes, jewel tones of green, purple or midnight blue work nicely.

*

There's nothing wrong with dewy skin as long as you avoid shimmer. Highlight cheekbones with a powder and steer clear of creamy highlighters.

PROFILE
SALINA THIND

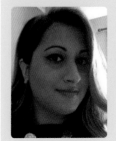
Salina Thind is a makeup artist and hair stylist with ten years' experience working in fashion, editorial, advertising and red carpet. Her celeb clients have included Gillian Anderson and Davina McCall. Salina is also beauty editor of *Fiasco* magazine.

Brights

Using bright shadows or liners can really make eyes 'pop'. For an on-trend effect, stick to matt powders, as shimmery brights can easily look garish and will age the face. As with a smoky or metallic eye, in order to let the standout feature shine, it's usually best to team bright eyes with a pared back lip colour such as nude or soft pink.

With brights, sometimes less is more. Sweeping a bright colour across the whole lid and up to the browbone can make you look like a five-year-old who has raided her mum's makeup bag. Try experimenting with a bright shadow below the crease of the eyelid only first, building up the colour slowly. Alternatively, use a bright liquid liner to create a thick feline flick across the top lid. Bright shadows look great with a clean, fine liner, or alone with lashings of black mascara. Just avoid the smudgy, smoky liner over a bright shadow, as the look will get messy and the impact of the colour will be lost.

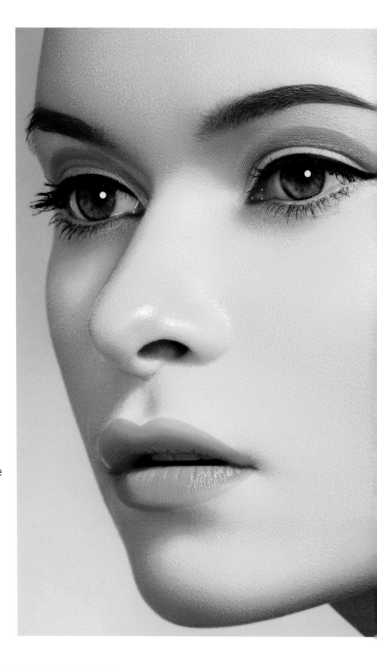

Pro's tip

For an even bolder effect or to brighten up a more softly pigmented shadow, use white eye pencil over the lid to create a base. This will make any shadow colour look stronger.

PROFILE
EMA DOHERTY

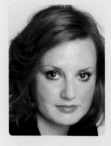

Ema Doherty has done makeup for TV and fashion shoots and been a judge for makeup competitions on television and at the Professional Beauty Awards. Ema has taught media, theatrical, camouflage, bridal and photographic makeup workshops in America, China, Russia and Monaco.

EMA DOHERTY'S STEP-BY-STEP GUIDE TO STANDOUT NEON EYES

1. Having chosen to make bright matt eyes the standout feature, first create contrast in your base by applying a dewy foundation to the skin. Pay particular attention to highlighting the cheekbone and browbone so that the eyes will be accented.

2. Use a subtle blush and a neutral tone on the lips, with a touch of shine to create a distinct contrast to the matt of the bright eyes.

3. Use a matt neon yellow powder as a shader by applying it to the eyelid. Blend it into the outer socket with a soft edge.

4. To create highlight, extend the yellow into the inner browbone, but this time leave a sharp edge rather than blending. This helps to prevent the effect looking flat.

5. Frame the bright eyes by using a dark brow powder to add definition to the brows.

6. Spike the lashes with dark black mascara, sectioning the lashline into five and clubbing each section together with wet mascara to form peaks. This mirrors the sharp, clean line of the neon yellow. As an alternative, spiky strip lashes could be applied.

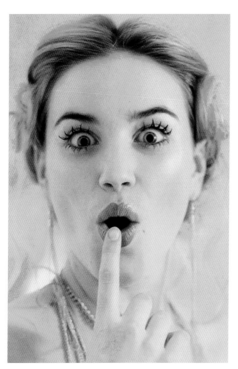

A 90s rave-inspired, neon-bright look by Ema Doherty

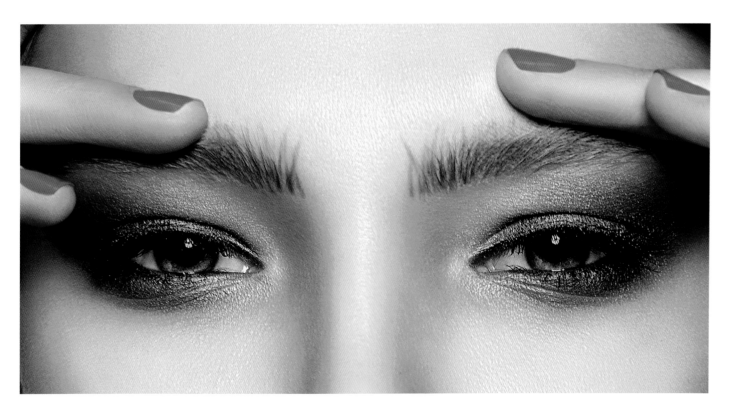

The feline flick

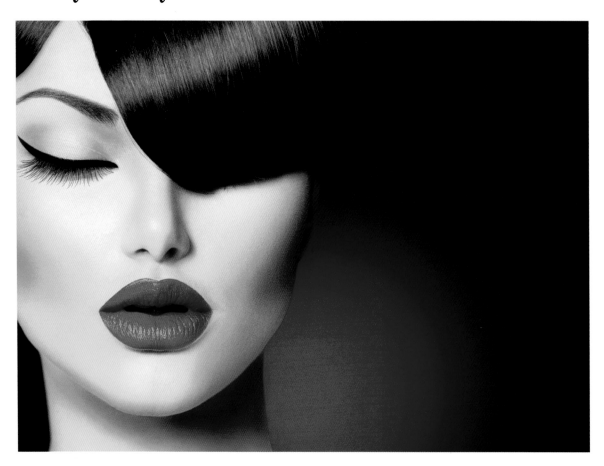

PERFECTING THE FLICK

The eyeliner flick gives a dramatic effect that works fantastically on its own, but can also add definition to a smoky eye or bright eyeshadow look. It bulks up the look of your lashes and is really versatile. Use the liner thin to create a sharp, sophisticated line for that Hollywood glamour effect, build it up thick for an edgy, rock chick look or go punky with extra length.

Liquid liner can be tricky to apply, especially if you don't have a steady hand, so look for one with a fine felt tip. Daniel Sandler recommends DHC liquid eyeliner. Once you've mastered the effect, try a liquid with a fine dip brush to achieve an even crisper line that won't fade or smudge. Benefit's Magic Ink is great for steadier hands.

PROFILE
DANIEL SANDLER

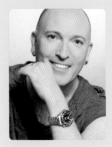

Daniel Sandler has worked on high-profile shoots and backstage at fashion shows for names such as Tom Ford and Tommy Hilfiger. But his real passion lies in making his stunning looks wearable for real women, showing them how easy makeup can be. He has his own range called Daniel Sandler Professional Finish Makeup.

DANIEL SANDLER'S STEP-BY-STEP GUIDE TO THE FELINE FLICK

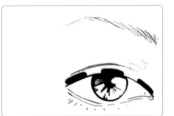

1. Take the liner as close as you can to the lashline. If you can't do the line all in one go, place shorter lines in each corner and one in the middle and join them up into a super-smooth line.

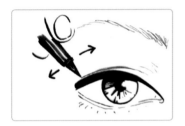

2. Use this line as a template to go backwards and forwards and build it up, taking the pen all the way from the inner to the outer corner.

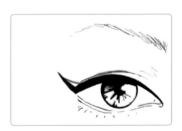

3. To create the flick, my guide is always to draw as if I'm continuing the line of the lower lashes, then flick up.

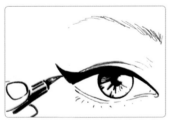

4. You can fill in any angles left between the main line and the flick by going backwards and forwards with the pen.

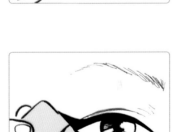

5. If you have trouble keeping the flick even, try using a credit card as a template, pressing it against your face at the desired angle. Repeat on the other eye so that the flicks are the same.

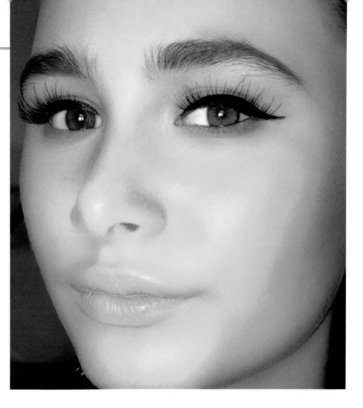

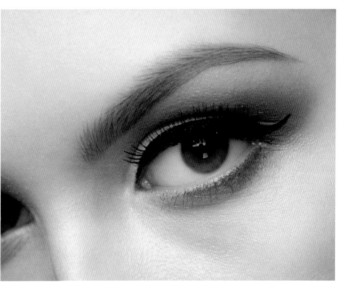

Liquid, gel or fibre-tipped eyeliners are perfect for the feline flick because they allow for a precise stroke. Fibre-tipped liners are easier to master as it's just like using a marker pen. But if you can get the hang of liquid or gel liners they allow you to create a very fine, crisp line and the ink will never bleed.

Pro's tip

If your line is uneven, use a makeup corrector pen or pointed cotton bud dipped in non-oily makeup remover to smooth it out, then reapply the liner.

Graphic eyeliner

The graphic eyeliner trend began on the catwalks at London Fashion Week and has been picked up by makeup artists across the UK. Black liquid liner with a very fine brush is your best bet for this technique, although a flat brush and gel liner will work well for some styles.

TAMARA TOTT'S TECHNIQUES FOR GRAPHIC LINER

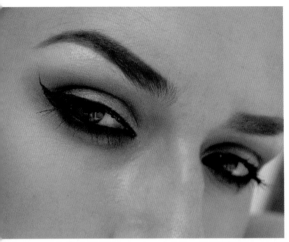

Dot and connect

This is a great technique for making sure both eyes are even. Use a liquid liner – Rimmel's has the thinnest brush I've seen so is great for precision. Tilt your head back and hold a mirror low so that your eyes are looking down.

Make a controlled dot where you want your graphic shape or line to finish. Draw a fine line to connect the outer corner of the eye with the dot. If drawing a flick, drag another line above the first line from the dot back to the corner of the eye to create a point. Then draw another line from the inner corner of the eye along the whole lid, keeping very close to the lash line. Gradually thicken this line to connect it smoothly to the flick.

Brush strokes

A flat, angled brush such as MAC 263 is great for creating a real cat's eye shape with an inner point as well as an outer flick, because its thin angle can get right into the inner corner of the eye. Use it with a gel eyeliner to create the lower line of the flick, then carefully sweep the line inwards from the flick along the whole lashline. Take the brush right into the inner corner of the eye, creating a thin line first then only thickening up if needed afterwards.

Shadow guide

Try drawing the shape you want with eyeshadow first. This way, if you make a mistake it's far less messy to remove and start again. Use an angled brush and a dark shadow to create your winged shape, then join it with the rest of the eye. When you have a look you like, go over it with liquid eyeliner.

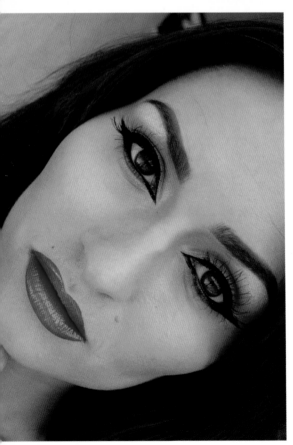

Use a gel liner and flat brush for this cat's eye look

PROFILE
TAMARA TOTT

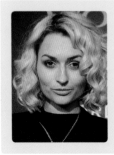

Tamara Tott is a freelance fashion and beauty makeup artist. In 2015 she won the Professional Beauty Makeup Specialist of the Year Award.

Powder stencil

Use a flat brush and some translucent powder to create a line in the direction you want your eyeliner to go. Then, with a liquid liner, make a dot where you want the line to finish, connect the line to the corner of the eye and fill. Tracing along the white powder will help you keep the liner straight. Once the liner is completely dry, use a fan brush to dust off the powder.

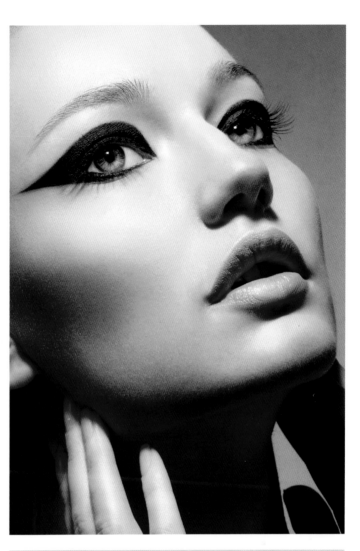

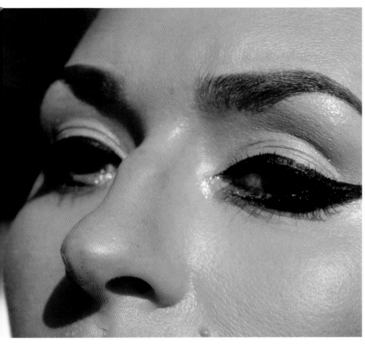

If you don't want to go for the full cat's eye, leave the inner corner open and thicken the lower line to create a broader wing

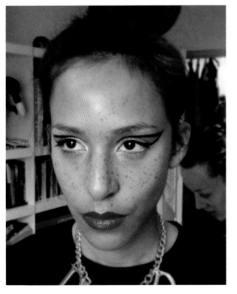

Left: the dot and connect technique is great for creating this outline flick

Right: once you've mastered basic graphic techniques, experiment with fine lines and dots

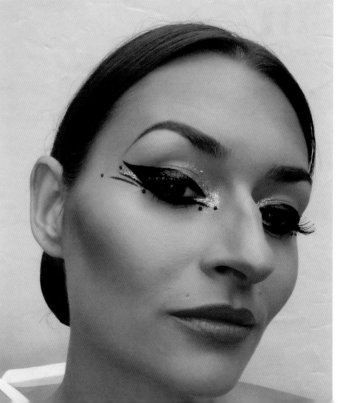

Luscious lashes

Enhancing the lashes is the quickest way to open up the eye area. Whether you reach for the mascara, stick on the strip lashes or go all out with professional extensions, creating longer, thicker lashes makes the eyes appear larger, younger and more feminine. Here pro MUA Karen Beadle shares her tips on choosing and applying the right look for you.

APPLYING MASCARA

Mascara is all about experimenting to find one that suits you. Use lash curlers to curl the top lashes, then add colour to the bottom lashes first. This avoids getting mascara stains on the top lids when you look up to coat the bottom lashes. Apply two or three coats for a fuller effect.

If you use mascara on a regular basis, be sure to use a lash conditioner or treatment. Overuse of some mascaras can make lashes brittle and cause them to break, so it's also a good idea to use a gentle eye makeup remover to dissolve your mascara.

Some mascaras have better brushes than others. Look for wands with a healthy, full brush that is slightly curved. This will help you catch all the lashes and encourage them to move in an upwards direction. It's often the brush rather than the mascara formula that makes the difference to the effect around the eyes. There are some great disposable mascara wands available.

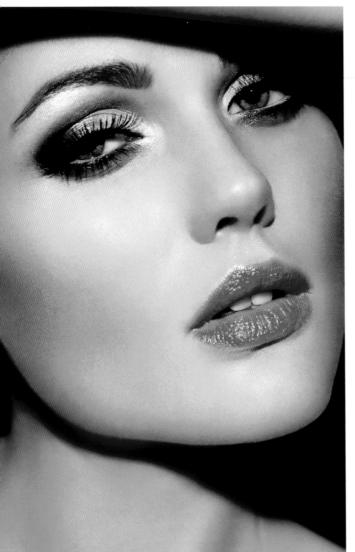

CHOOSING FALSE LASHES

There are three main styles of false lash: strip, corner or individual lashes. Whichever you choose, make sure they are not too long or thick, especially if you have deep-set eyes, as they will look theatrical and doll-like.

When choosing strip lashes, go a touch longer or the same length as your natural lashes and look for a strip that matches the width of your eyelid. Be wary of cutting them down as it can ruin the shape. A safer bet is to buy corner lashes. These are short strips that enhance the outside edge of your eye and will blend in with your real lashes.

For an even more natural look, individual lashes often come in small clusters and can be used along the outside half of the lashline.

PROFILE
KAREN BEADLE

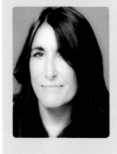

Karen Beadle is a celebrity makeup artist with a background in fashion photography, beauty, film and music. As a beauty editor and writer, she writes about trends in skincare and makeup and runs makeup courses. Her expertise extends to bridal and red carpet events and her clients include Thandi Newton and Julie Walters.

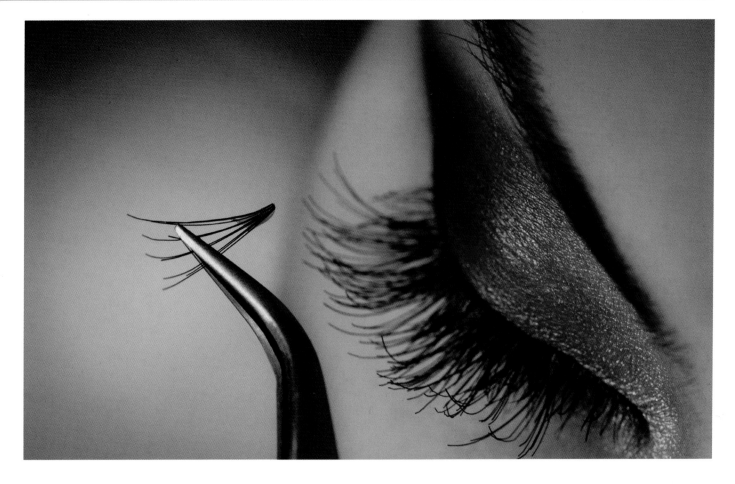

APPLYING INDIVIDUAL LASHES

These come in medium and longer lengths and it's a good idea to mix the two for a more natural effect, using the longer lengths at the outside edges only. Squeeze a little glue onto the back of the lash packet then pick up one lash and dip the base in the glue before placing it carefully on top of your natural lashes where they grow from the lid.

KAREN BEADLE'S STEP-BY-STEP TO APPLYING STRIP LASHES

1. Using tweezers, unglue the lashes carefully from the packaging and place onto the back of your hand.

2. Take a lash glue and spread the applicator along the underside of the lash.

3. Bring the lash up to your eye, making sure the shortest length is in the corner near your nose. Starting at that inside edge, place the strip on the line where the lid meets the lashes, making sure it fits neatly into the corner, and along the full lashline.

4. Wait about 30 seconds for the glue to dry, then open your eyes.

5. If the lashes comes unstuck, add a bit of the lash glue to the tip of pointed tweezers, then carefully apply it under the lash and stick it back down.

Pro's tip

For a dramatic look, try curling false lashes and adding a small amount of mascara to them before applying.

Defined brows

Full, heavily defined brows are really on trend, thanks to catwalk models such as Cara Delevingne, and these styles can easily be created at home. The key to getting the full brow look right is keeping the hair long and textured while still maintaining a structured shape. Take away too much of the natural hair and you'll have to draw in the shape, which will end up looking fake and harsh.

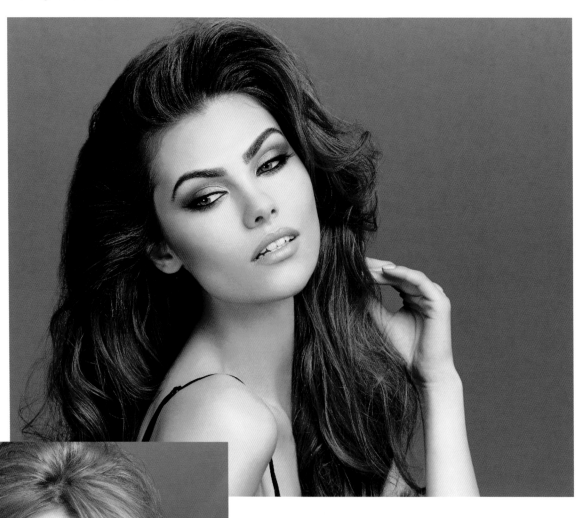

PROFILE
NILAM HOLMES-PATEL

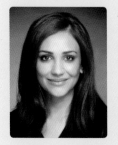

As founder of HD Brows, Nilam Holmes-Patel is responsible for bringing the power brow from the catwalk to the masses. Her work can be seen in music videos, movies and TV commercials around the world. With a portfolio of A-list clients, Nilam is the celebs' go-to girl for brow styling advice.

NILAM HOLMES-PATEL'S STEP-BY-STEP TO BEAUTIFUL BROWS

1. Use a brow pencil to draw in the shape of the brows, incorporating as much of your own hair as possible. Try using a brow stencil as a guide to make sure you get an even shape on both sides.

2. Tweeze away the hairs outside the shape you've drawn, to keep the brow tidy. Avoid taking away any hairs from the body of the brow or you'll risk losing the shape.

3. Master the use of a brow pencil so that you can mimic super-fine hair strokes and fill in any sparse areas. To do this, always draw light strokes in the direction of the hair growth, ensuring lines are clean and accurate. Opt for a brow pencil enriched with waxes for optimum texture, as these are ideal to fill, define and shape the eyebrows to perfection.

4. For a bolder look, use a brow powder to quickly fill in any spaces in the brows. Apply it with an angled brush to create a fuller look.

5. Once you have the desired shape and definition, use a brush-on tinted brow gel to set your brows in place without flaking or stiffening the hair. Use one with a tapered applicator wand to make it super-easy to apply. These offer a professional, well-groomed finish that can fix your brows in place, ensuring they look great from desk to disco!

Pro's tips

Make sure you match your brow colour to your skin tone. Blondes should go one to two shades darker than their natural hair colour, and brunettes should go one to two shades lighter.

*

If you haven't got much brow hair, don't worry. Products such as a nourishing serum or gel packed full of powerful ingredients can be used to speed up the hair growth.

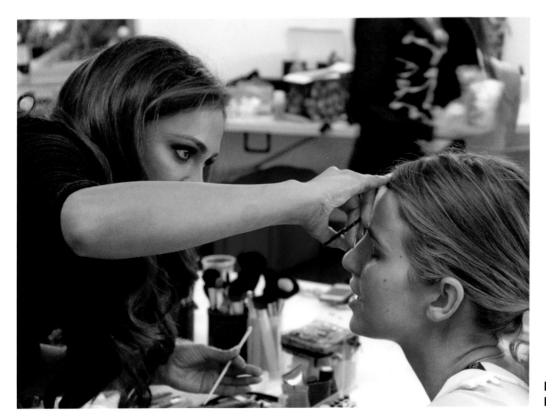

Defined brows by Nilam Holmes-Patel using HD Brows products

Makeup for glasses wearers

Glasses draw attention to the eye area, so if you wear them practise creating some works of art to put inside those frames. There is a huge variety of specs frames available and investing in more than one pair gives you the freedom to experiment with shadow and lipstick shades to complement them – or to deliberately clash with them for a high-impact look. Different lens prescriptions can affect the appearance of the eyes, so you may need to adjust your makeup if your prescription changes. Glasses can also create shine or indentations where they touch the skin, so try some of these tips from glasses-wearing pro makeup artist Armand Beasley to keep the oil to a minimum and makeup in place all day long.

ARMAND BEASLEY'S TIPS FOR GLASSES WEARERS

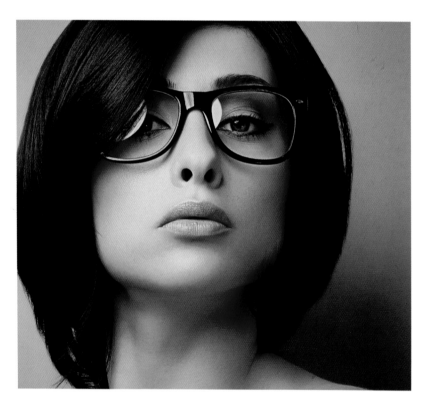

1. Add silver or gold to the inner corner of your eyes to help brighten them. Sisley and MAC both have gorgeous shimmer shadows that will brighten without looking glittery.

2. If you are short-sighted your prescription will make your eyes look smaller. To counteract this, invest in a soft, white liner to use along the waterline. NARS Larger Than Life Long-Wear Eyeliner in Santa Monica Blvd or Avon SuperShock Gel Eyeliner Pencil in silver are perfect.

3. If you are long-sighted your lenses will make your eyes look bigger, so go for a smoky eye. You can get away with lots of black liner, even inside the waterline, to bring a bit of drama to the eyes.

4. Don't be lazy with your brows. A good eyebrow shape not only adds polish to your look, but can also take years off you.

5. Don't be scared of colour clash. If you have a bold specs frame colour like orange, try clashing it with a fuchsia-pink lip.

6. Wearing glasses, especially ones with a heavy frame, can generate more oil production around the eyes, which means shadow will crease quickly. Combat this by

PROFILE
ARMAND BEASLEY

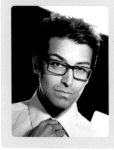

Armand Beasley has worked on events ranging from the Oscars to the BAFTAs and with actors such as Goldie Hawn and Michelle Keegan. He has worked as UK national makeup artist for Givenchy and done makeup for editorial features in *Grazia*, *Hello* and *Fabulous* magazines.

using an eyeshadow primer such as NARS Smudge Proof Eyeshadow Base before applying powder shadows, then spritz with a makeup setting spray afterwards.

7. With larger frames there's a bigger spotlight for eye makeup, so practise those feline liner flicks.

8. If you get annoyed with the little dents that your frames leave on the bridge of your nose, invest in a makeup primer to help keep your foundation in place, then layer with an oil-free foundation down the T-zone. Use a shine-control powder such as MAC's Blot Powder to minimize the marks; it will absorb excess oil without caking you in makeup.

9. Bring out your eye colour by using contrasting shadows. If you have blue eyes, try green; if your eyes are green, try purple; and if they're brown, experiment with blue shades.

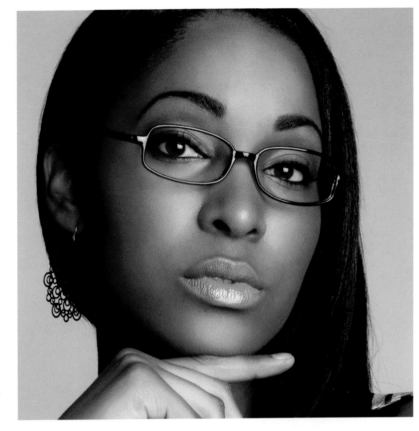

Pro's tips

If you have standout fashion frames, try keeping eyeshadow colours neutral to let the frames do the talking. Then add pops of colour on the lips or cheeks.

If you wear thick frames, use a thicker stroke of liquid eyeliner to balance them.

Dark circles can be accentuated by glasses. Brighten the area under your eye with an illuminating concealer or powder.

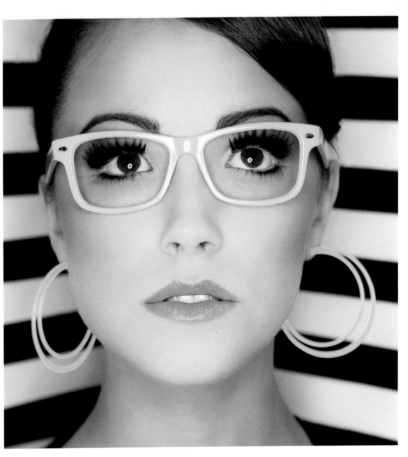

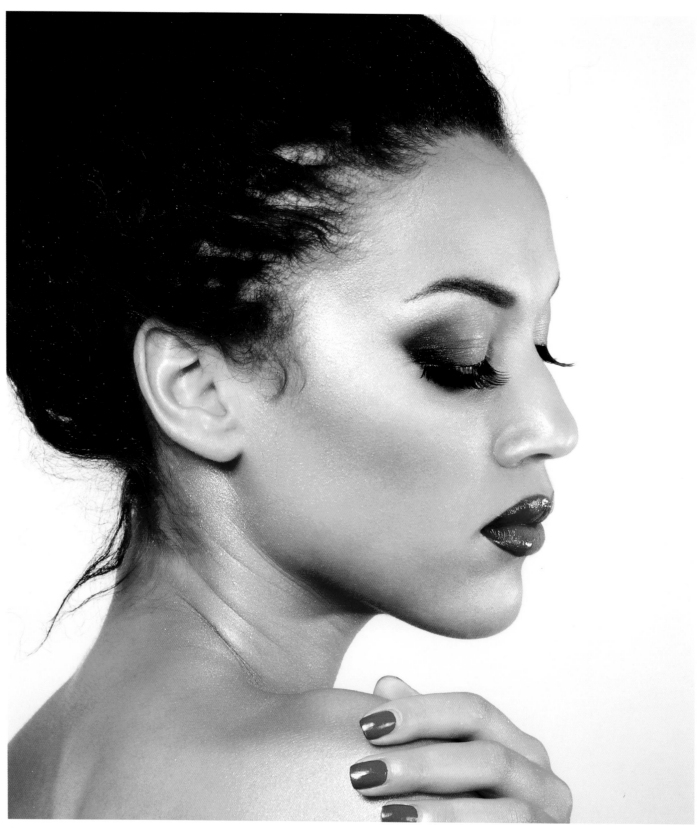

A highly contoured makeup look finished with super-glossy lips

Chapter Four

Contours and Kisses

A flush of colour on the cheeks and lips can transform your face, lifting your complexion and breathing radiance into a tired makeup look.

Blusher can also help to change the shape of your face. Combine it with shadow and highlighter to contour, creating the illusion of great bone structure, or buff gently into the apples of the cheeks for a youthful rosy glow that softens your whole look. You can also use blusher to widen a long face shape or slim down a round face with careful placement and blending.

Bronzer is another tool that can take you from washed out to warm glow in the sweep of a brush, but it's one that is easy to get wrong. Shun the high-shimmer and orange-hued bronzers of old and embrace a subtle sunkiss with some application tips from the pros. You can also use matt bronzer to create super-soft shadows that tighten up the jawline, shorten the nose or enhance the swell of the lips.

When it comes to the lips themselves, look beyond the lipstick and switch up your routine with lip stains, pencils, glosses, powders and highlighters to create lasting block colour, or cheat pumped-up volume. Learn from the top makeup artists about layering product to keep colour in place all day long and experiment with new shades to complement your colouring.

Choosing and applying blusher

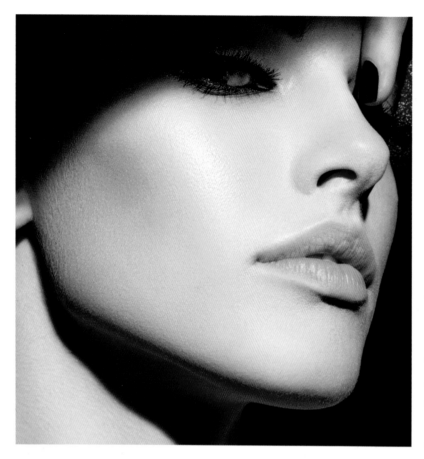

Applied correctly, blusher can slim your face, accentuate your cheekbones and give a radiant glow. As with all makeup, playing around with different colours, textures and positioning is the best way to find what works for you. While general guidelines say baby pink suits fair skin, breaking the rules with a hit of hot pink can make a real impact and offset a super-bright lipstick. Using a few pro tips as a starting point, you can quickly get to know the shades and formulations that will create the look you want.

COLOUR MATCH

With dark skin tones, blush can sometimes melt into the skin with poor colour payoff, so use shades that look brighter than you want in the palette, then build up slowly. Red and orange-based pinks work well, but give deeper plum shades a try, too, for a natural lift.

Medium skin tones should use peach and coral shades for the most natural effect, but look out for raspberry or brown-based pinks for a stronger finish. If you have medium skin with a cooler undertone, hot pink applied sheer looks pretty.

Fair skins can work soft pinks well for that English rose effect, but peach, which has both pink and yellow undertones, will also look good, especially if your pale skin has warm undertones. If you do opt for brights, build up colour gradually and blend well.

Pro's tip

For a natural glowing look, apply cream blusher before your foundation so that it shines through. Finish with a light application of powder blush to accentuate.

TEXTURE CHOICE

Powder works on most skins, but is particularly good for oilier types. Apply over base powder so that it blends smoothly and builds colour, or use wet for a bolder colour pay-off.

Cream blush is great for dry skins as it is hydrating and blends easily. Many makeup artists find it gives a more natural glow and lasts better than powder. Try layering cream and powder for even longer wear.

Liquid formulations are designed to give a watercolour effect and blend seamlessly. Apply a few drops with a flat brush and blend well. They work best on well-hydrated or oily skins.

GET IN SHAPE

Natural glow For a soft finish that suits any face shape, buff the blush into the apples of your cheeks with a soft round brush, blending out slightly along the cheekbone. For a more dramatic effect, blend upwards towards the temples and into your hairline.

For long faces Keep the blush to the apples of the cheeks, blending in wider circles. Take it back just slightly towards the temple, but not to the hairline. This gives the illusion of width.

For round faces Feel for your cheekbones then apply the blusher just where the hollow of your cheeks meets the bottom of the bone. Blend in a straight line upwards to the temple and into the hair. This is a similar trick to contouring, but quicker and with a softer effect.

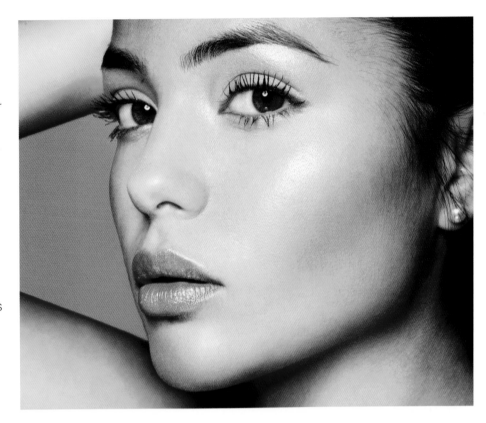

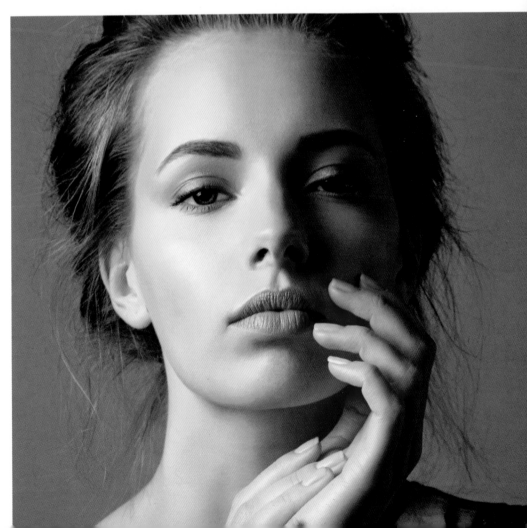

Contouring with powder

In essence, contouring uses dark colours to make things look further away and light colours and shimmers to bring them nearer. It can be done with liquid foundation and highlighters, but you can also use powder formulations either instead of liquids for a softer effect or on top to set the liquid shading formulas and add extra shadow and light at the end. To contour with powder, set your foundation with loose powder first to create a dry base.

TOOLS TO CONTOUR

- A matt bronzer or eyeshadow two to three shades darker than your skin.
- A slanted blusher brush or specialist contouring brush. 'These are square to give a really sharp line. I use one by Royal & Langnickel,' says pro MUA Anne Bowcock.
- A softer, small, tapered brush to contour around the hairline, such as Real Techniques bronzer/blusher brush.

TOOLS TO HIGHLIGHT

- Shimmer highlighting powder or eyeshadow. Golden tones work well on dark skins and pale pearlescents on light skins.
- A small, fluffy brush. If your brush is too big it will take the highlighting outside the area and ruin the rest of your makeup.

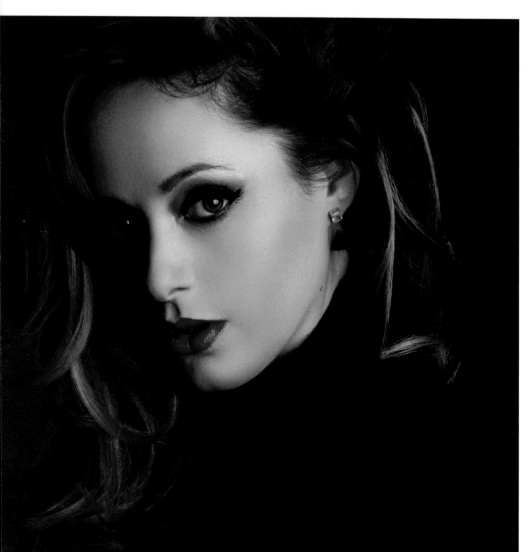

Pro's tip

Keep old eyeshadows: bash the dark ones together to create contour powder and do the same with the light ones for highlighter. Shimmer shadows are fine for highlighting, but not for contouring powder, as they will bring out an area rather than disguise it.

A strong, contoured look by Anne Bowcock as part of an ad campaign for fashion label Harlem Carter

ANNE BOWCOCK'S STEP-BY-STEP GUIDE TO CONTOURING WITH POWDER

1. Feel around your cheekbones so you know where you want to shade. Start from the middle of the ear and shade down diagonally below the cheekbone.

2. Shade the forehead depending on your hair growth. If your hairline is set far back, shade the top of the forehead to lessen that. If you have a lot of hair around the temples, don't shade too much here as it will make your forehead look narrow. Blend the powder down to the temples, not over the whole face.

3. Shade down the sides of the nose. You can also shade below the tip of the nose. If you have a long nose, shade just above the tip as well to shorten the appearance.

4. The ideal face shape is oval – anything else you need to balance. So if you have a square jaw, shade each side to make it look tapered. For jowly areas, shade the skin where it covers the jaw then blend backwards. If you have a double chin, shade out that whole area.

5. To highlight, brush your shimmer powder along the very top of the cheekbone and diagonally up into the temples. Don't take the shimmer into the eye area, where skin starts to get thinner.

6. Highlight along the centre of the nose. If your nose is long, stop before you get to the area you shaded earlier. Take the shimmer up from the bridge of the nose above the brows, gently blending to fan it out over the brows in an arch.

7. Highlighting the Cupid's bow is great for thinner lips to give the illusion of fullness. Highlighting around the corners of the mouth lifts and makes for a brighter smile. But be careful on older skin as it will emphasize any fine lines. Add light to the centre of the chin and anywhere else that would naturally catch the light, where the bones should protrude.

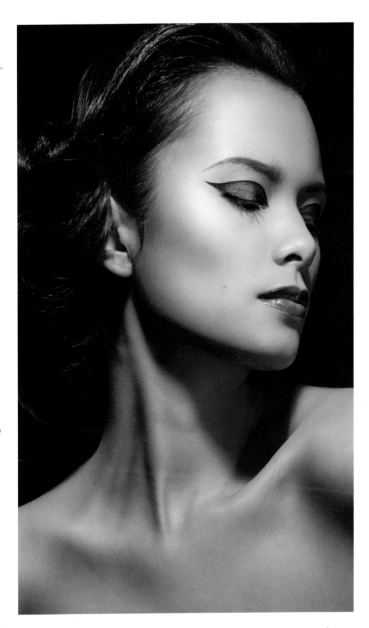

PROFILE
ANNE BOWCOCK

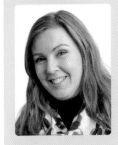

Anne Bowcock is head of makeup artistry for ADCreativ and often runs a team of artists at red carpet events. She has also had her work featured in national magazines. She is now fulfilling her dream with a teaching career, inspiring the next generation of makeup artists.

Creating fuller lips

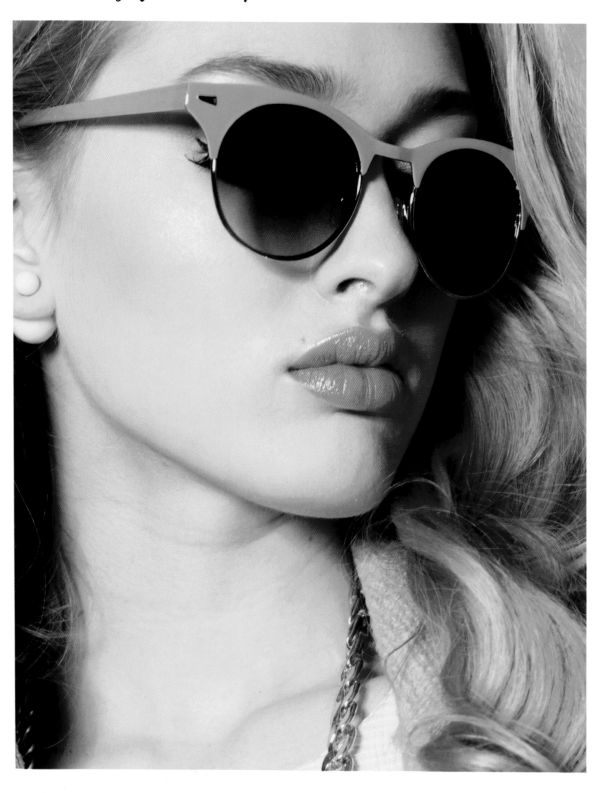

We all long for a luscious bee-stung pout, but full lips such as this only seem to come naturally to the likes of Scarlett Johansson and Angelina Jolie. As we age, the lips get thinner and the top part of the upper lip – known as the Cupid's bow – begins to flatten, making the pout less pronounced. But there are a few tricks which can help you create the illusion of youthful fullness and depth.

KAREN BEADLE'S STEP-BY-STEP GUIDE TO CREATING FULLER-LOOKING LIPS

1. Dryness or dehydration will make lips look smaller, so start by exfoliating and moisturizing. Apply a little lip balm during preparation, but make sure the lip is clean and dry with no oils before you begin applying colour.

2. Some lip colours look better with a lip primer underneath, which helps to show the true pigment of strong colours and prevents bleeding over the lipline.

3. It's better to use light, translucent lip colours to create a fuller mouth. If the colour is too creamy or too matt it will flatten the look of the lip, making it look smaller and too harsh.

4. Use a good, pointed lip brush and apply a clean line to the outside of the lips. Smooth the colour over the shape of your lips and carefully into the corner of the mouth very cleanly, making sure it stays just within the lipline.

5. Take a sharp lip pencil around the same tone or a touch darker than your lipstick colour and draw lightly around and slightly over the lipline to sharpen and improve the shape.

6. Use a lip highlighter or lip maximizer over the Cupid's bow to give the illusion of depth.

7. Finally, blend the outer line into the skin around the outside of the lip for a softer finish.

Pro's tips

Try adding a slightly brighter colour to the centre of the lips to help create a more 3D effect, but keep it subtle and be sure to blend it well.

*

Taking bright colour outside the natural lipline looks fake. If your lips are unbalanced, use a neutral-toned lip pencil to even them out. Buff the colour on using small strokes. Start inside the lip then gradually push the boundary out slightly. Don't go too far beyond the natural colour, just boost it slightly in any uneven areas and never go higher on the Cupid's bow.

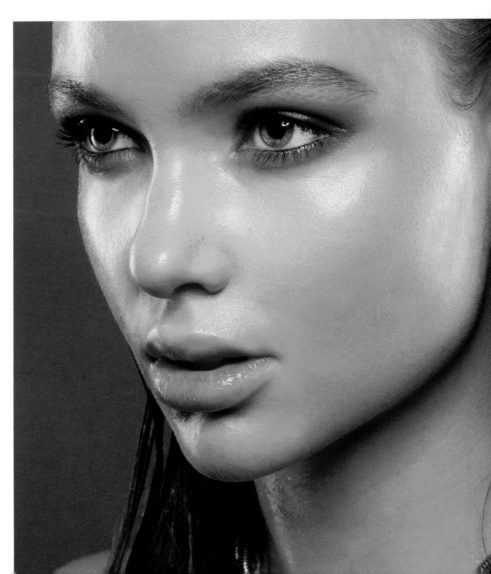

The perfect red lip

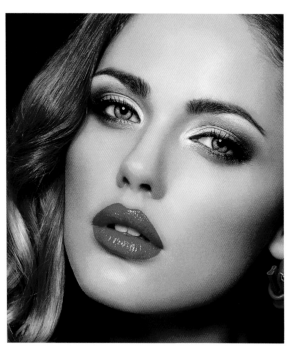

Bright red lipstick certainly makes a statement and many women use it as part of a strong signature look. Red lips can look classy or vintage, and they can also be very cool. Once you've mastered the technique to achieve a flawless finish with staying power, the red lip can be a fantastic way to add a touch of glamour to any makeup look. Pair it with a simple slick of mascara to let the lips do all the talking or go bold by teaming it with a smoky eye for high-impact evening glamour.

The most important parts of the process are prep and layering because if you just grab a red lipstick and apply it from the bullet, expecting it to stay put, it won't and you'll end up with smudges all over your face and faded patches where the lips meet.

A hot red lip against a flawless base, styled by Sothys makeup artists

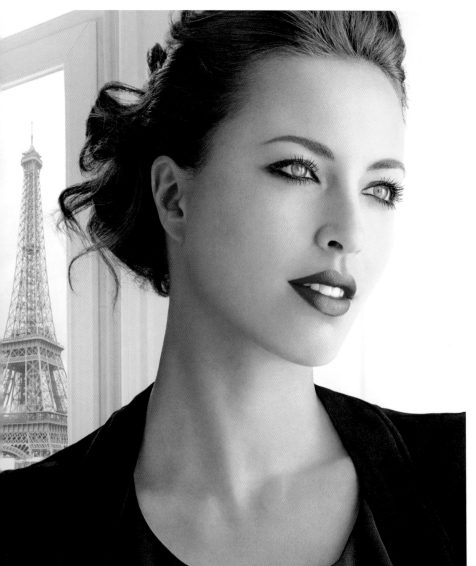

Pro's tip

If you have problems keeping the colour firmly in place, look out for the two-step lip products that have a liquid colour at one end and a sealing balm at the other. They really do stain your lips and keep the colour solid.

AIMEE ADAMS'S STEP-BY-STEP GUIDE TO THE PERFECT RED LIP

1. If there is any dryness or flakiness, red lipstick will look terrible, so start by gently exfoliating with a lip scuff or sugar scrub – or even by gently rubbing with a toothbrush or flannel.

2. To carry off a red lip, you need to think of the rest of the face first. If you have any other redness such as a red vein on the nose or any spots, red lipstick will emphasize it, so cover these areas with a good concealer or foundation first. You can also use a nude pencil around the inside of the eye so the only red on the face will be the lips.

3. You can buy the most expensive lipstick brand in the world, but if you don't prep the base properly it will still shift in ten minutes as soon as you eat or drink. Apply concealer or highlighter around the lips and right up to the lipline to prevent the colour bleeding. Some makeup artists apply base, but I prefer not to.

4. Use a lip stain to create a base colour on the lip, so if some of the lipstick colour does rub off you still have some colour beneath. Stains come in a felt tip-style pen and are better for a base than a pencil because they really do stain the lip and don't slide off.

5. Next take a lip pencil. I like Rimmel's 1000 Kisses because it has great staying power. Sketch in the shape of your lips. Do it in a magnifying mirror for precision, then step back and look at the shape in a normal mirror to check that it's even.

6. Apply the lipstick. You can do this with a brush or straight from the bullet. A brush will give a more precise line. Blot with a tissue. Apply a very fine layer of loose translucent powder, such as Corn Silk Powder. Apply a second layer of lipstick colour and blot and powder a second time to set the colour.

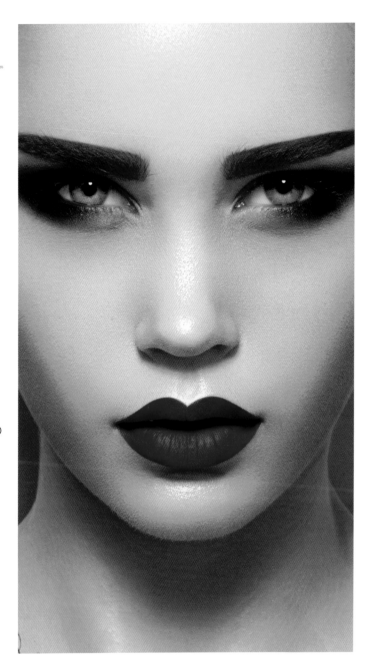

PROFILE
AIMEE ADAMS

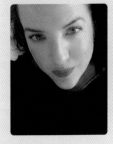

Aimee Adams is a makeup artist to the stars. Her client list includes pop legends such as Madonna and supermodels such as Erin O'Connor. She spends much of her time travelling the world on editorial shoots for major glossies such as *Vogue*, *Elle* and *Marie Claire*.

Personalizing the red lip

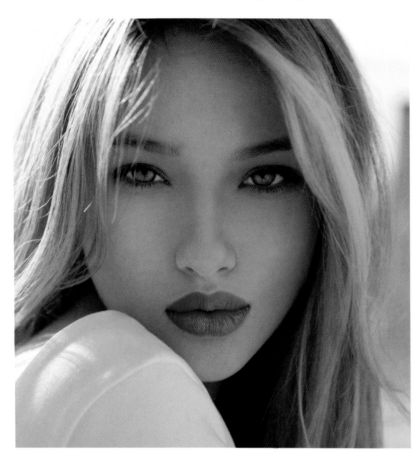

A bright red lip can be scary. Many people think of them as vampy or daring, but there are lots of things you can do to dip your toe in the water and try out a subtle red look without going all out. Likewise, there are lots of tips and tricks to choosing the right shade and texture of red to complement your skin tone and the rest of your makeup.

KEEPING RED SUBTLE

Try applying the lipstick with your middle finger, dabbing it on lightly, rather than using a brush or applying from the tube. This will keep the colour softer and give it more of a matt finish. Blend it in with a cotton bud to create a soft, stained effect. Build up colour gradually in layers for a stronger look without that polished finish.

CHOOSING THE RIGHT SHADE

Most people test lipsticks on the inside of the wrist or the back of the hand, but that doesn't give you a good idea of how the shade will look with your facial skin tone and the rest of your features.

A great way to test out shades in the shop before you buy is to apply the tester to your index and middle finger tips, then to hold your fingers in front of your lips as you look in the mirror. You may feel a bit silly, but you'll make fewer mistakes because you'll see at firsthand how the colour will work with the rest of your face.

There are certain 'rules' about which reds suit which skin tone, but you'll know instinctively whether a shade feels right for you or if it makes your teeth look yellow or deepens the dark circles under your eyes.

THE 'RULES'

Like all rules, these are meant to be broken and you should play around with lots of colours until you find some you like. Nevertheless, this guide gives a good starting point to choosing your go-to red.

The fairer your skin, hair and eyes, the more orangey or coral the shade you should choose.

If you have medium to dark skin or hair, opt for the more blue-based reds, such as those with a berry or plum tone.

Black women can carry off dark cherry shades very well, but hot pop colours like orange also look great against dark skin.

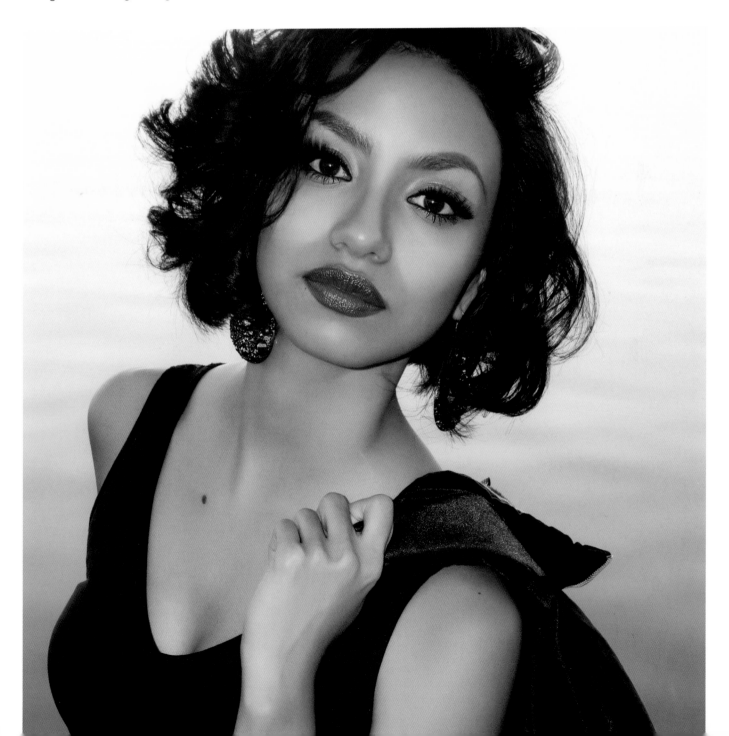

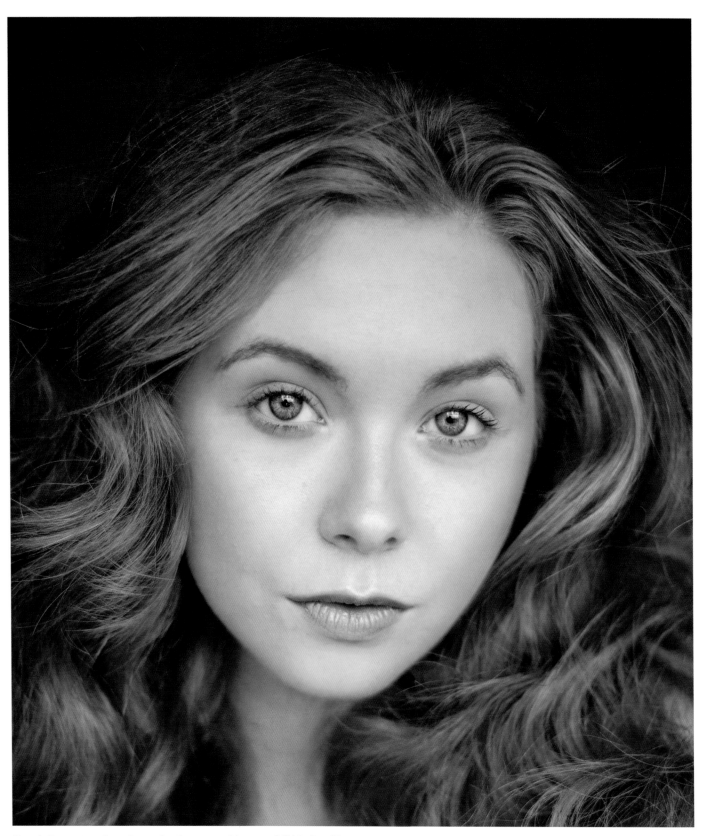

A subtle, natural makeup look created by pro MUA Jen Hunter

Chapter Five

Swift and Simple

A killer smoky eye and perfect contouring may be the things that drive your love of makeup, but most days you'll need a faster and subtler route to polished perfection. Whether it's speed or simplicity you're after – or both – there are plenty of tips and tricks for achieving everyday-fabulous makeup.

Most professionals agree that a low-key look starts with the skin, so getting the basics right is the best starting point, especially when you want to look like you haven't even tried. Establishing a fail-safe look for work or college means mastering some shortcuts so that you can be prepped and out of the door at speed. When time is tight, makeup multi-taskers come into their own, so keep an eye out for cheek and lip tints which can be used as blush, lipstick and even eyeshadow, at a push, and for BB and CC creams that provide the best quick cover-up.

Creating a capsule kit is also a great way to prep for makeup on the move, so seek out essentials with a dual function – long-wearing hero pieces and saviours that let you freshen up your look fast. You can look perfect, even when you are in a rush. Whether you have an hour to prep for a party, or just five minutes, this chapter contains the ultimate roundup of quick tricks and hot beauty shortcuts.

The capsule kit

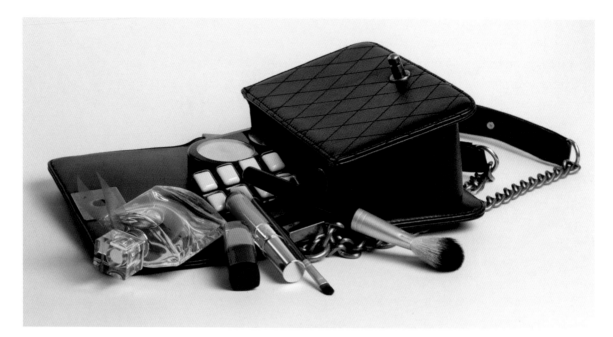

Most makeup lovers and all pro makeup artists will have a huge collection of products, but only a handful of firm favourites. However, sifting through to find the essentials to carry on a holiday, work trip or night out can still be a challenge. You want to be covered for every eventuality without having to lug around a bulging makeup bag that almost qualifies for the excess baggage fee by itself! By choosing some clever multi-taskers and keeping the concealer close at hand, you can create a wide range of looks and keep them fresh day to night.

FRANCESCA NEILL'S TIPS FOR PUTTING TOGETHER A CAPSULE KIT

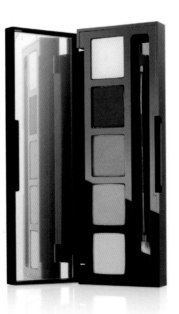

For a trip away
- good foundation or tinted moisturizer with SPF
- concealer
- bronzer
- cream blusher
- mascara
- nude eyeshadow palette
- brow pencil
- eyeliner
- lip gloss

This kit covers you for every occasion when you're away on a trip. You can create a natural 'no makeup makeup' look by simply applying cream blush onto cheeks for day, then adding more in the evening for a fresh, dewy look. All these products can take you from day to night.

For a day or night out

If you're going to be carrying a handbag around all day, you want to pack light. Choose multi-tasking products such as lip and cheek tints. These are brilliant, as they are the perfect size for travelling and can be used on cheeks, eyes, lips and even blended as eyeshadow. There are also some great versatile products for the eyes, such as the HD Brows Eye & Brow Palette, which can be used on brows, for shadow to create a smoky eye look, and even as eyeliner.

For an evening bag

When space is almost too tight for makeup, the main essential is concealer so that you can touch up throughout the night and keep your makeup looking fresh. If there's room, I also like to carry a bronzer and a lip gloss or balm to keep lips looking plump.

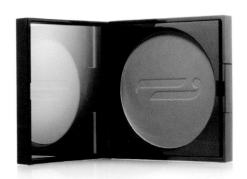

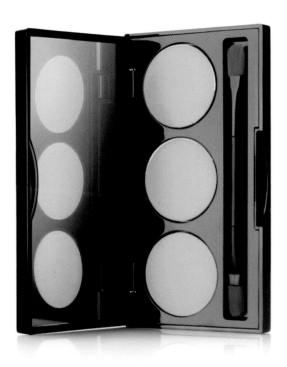

PROFILE
FRANCESCA NEILL

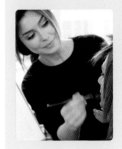

Francesca Neill is a celebrity makeup artist. She has worked with Alesha Dixon, Girls Aloud, Little Mix, Amanda Holden and Rochelle Humes, to name but a few, and she toured with Girls Aloud in 2013. Francesca is creative director for Makeup by HD Brows.

The 'no-makeup makeup' look

Creating natural makeup that looks as though you wake up every morning with flawless skin and bright eyes is a great skill. Perfecting that youthful 'drop dead gorgeous without even trying' image takes a great, illuminating base and some subtle tricks to open up the eyes and define the lips.

Natural, flawless, fresh makeup by Catherine Bailey

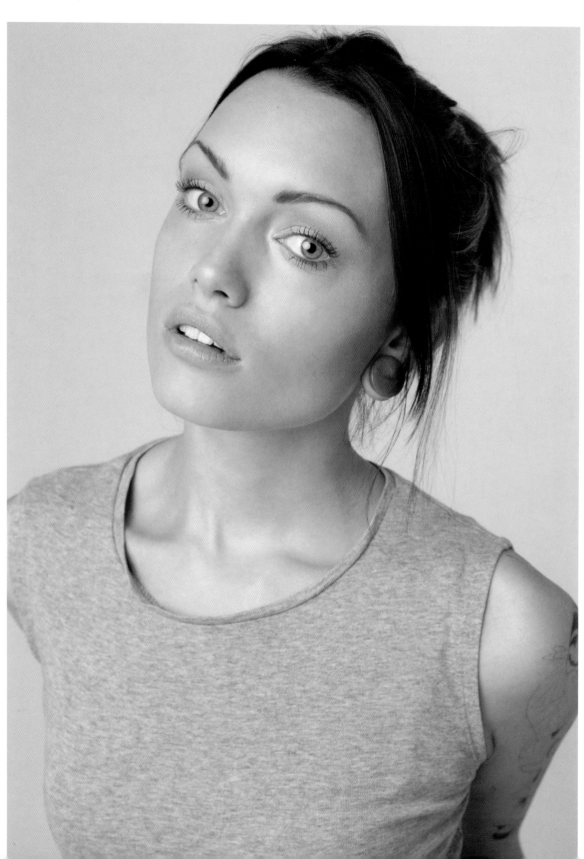

CATHERINE BAILEY'S STEP-BY-STEP GUIDE TO THE NO-MAKEUP MAKEUP LOOK

1. Apply a light, slightly dewy base, such as Liz Earle Sheer Skin Tint using a flat foundation brush, a damp sponge or your fingers.

2. Conceal under the eyes to get rid of dark circles, soften lines and ensure you look fresh and awake. Use a creamy concealer such as NARS Radiant Creamy Concealer rather than a powder or liquid, as this will give good coverage without looking too dry or heavy. Set your base with a sheer face powder.

3. Apply a matt ivory eyeshadow all over the lid to brighten, and then a matt taupe eyeshadow in the socket to add subtle definition.

4. Curl your lashes gently to make your eyes look more awake, then set with two fine coats of dark brown mascara. Brush a brow powder or brow mascara through your brows for natural definition.

5. Dab a sheer nude pink lipstick onto your lips with your fingers. I used Bobbi Brown's lipstick in Bare Pink.

6. Use a matching cream blusher on the apples of your cheeks and along the cheekbone, blending well for a natural finish.

Pro's tip

Perfecting the natural look is all about keeping the base light while ensuring good coverage, so skip the powders and stick to sheer liquids. If foundation looks too heavy, try a BB cream.

The 'no makeup makeup' look

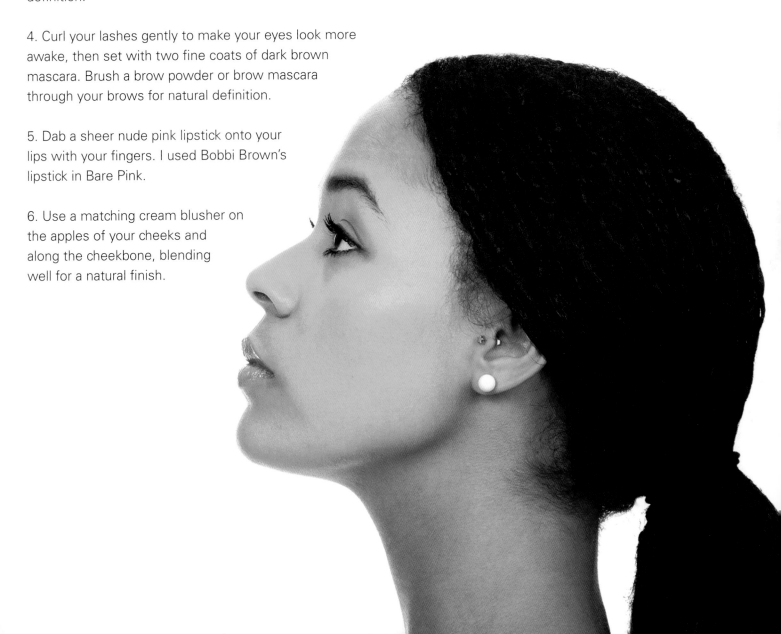

Workday fabulous

Getting office makeup right requires a delicate balance. You want to look groomed and polished, but not as though you're ready for a big night out. Above all, you still want to look like yourself.

When time is tight and you need to do your work makeup in a hurry, choose the three key products that make the biggest difference – mascara, blush and a hydrating nude lipstick.

Pro's tips

Look for long-lasting formulas when buying cream eyeshadows and lipsticks to minimize makeup touch-ups throughout the day.

✳

To refresh your makeup at work, invest in a spritz product such as MAC Prep + Prime Fix+. This hydrates the skin and stops your makeup looking tired later in the day.

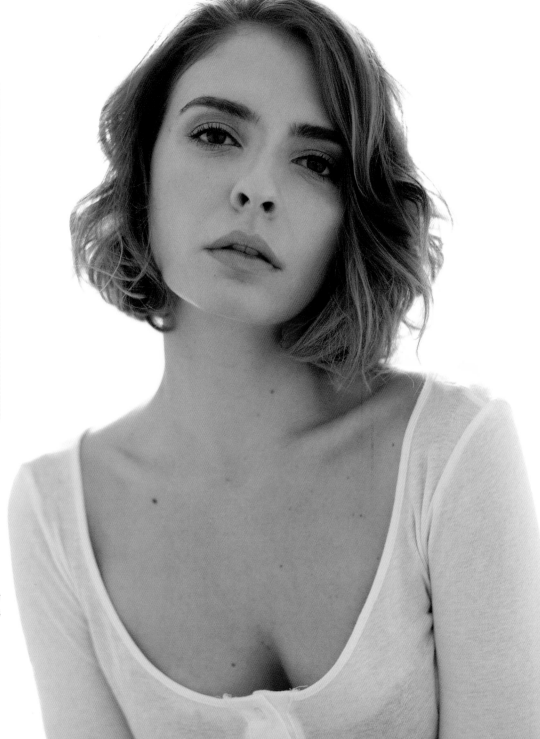

A subtle everyday look by Pamela Moss

PAMELA MOSS'S STEP-BY-STEP GUIDE TO SOFT, EVERYDAY WORK MAKEUP

1. Apply a liquid foundation or tinted moisturizer with your fingers or a brush. Liquid foundations blend easily and are more forgiving when you are in a hurry.

2. Conceal under the eyes with a light-reflecting pen such as Clinique's Airbrush Concealer pen. This will make you look wide-awake and ready for the day.

3. Use a brow pencil to groom brows and fill in any sparse areas. Well-groomed brows frame the eyes so it's worth spending the time on this.

4. For the eyes, apply a nude cream shadow all over the lid as a base. Cream shadows are great for longevity. Use a darker brown powder shadow in the outer corner of the eye and blend in along the socket line. Finish with black mascara on the top lashes to give your eyes subtle definition.

5. Apply a soft pink or peach powder blush to the apples of your cheeks and sweep upwards and outwards towards the temples – just enough to give you a healthy glow.

6. A nude lipstick will pull the look together and give it polish. For the days when you feel like making a statement, a soft red lipstick will add a pop of colour. You most certainly can wear red lipstick to the office – just leave eyes nude with mascara and little or no liner, to keep the look soft rather than vampy.

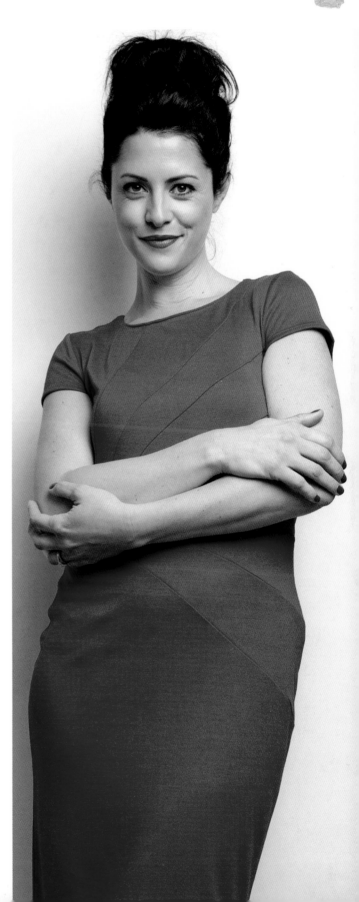

PROFILE
PAMELA MOSS

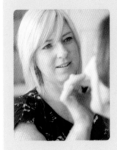

Pamela Moss began her career as a makeup artist for Yves Saint Laurent and has since gone on to work for clients including Bobbi Brown. Pamela is also the founder of Mode Makeup School, where she trains the next generation of makeup artists.

A striking professional makeup look by Pamela Moss

Ten-minute makeup

We've all pressed that snooze button once too often and been left making a mad dash to get out of the door for work. At times like this your usual routine won't cut it, so you need some time-saving makeup tricks up your sleeve. Invest in quick-to-apply, multi-tasking products such as BB cream, cheek and lip tint and cream eyeshadow and try the following fall-back look the next time you need to work some ten-minute magic.

TAMARA TOTT'S TEN-MINUTE MAKEUP LOOK

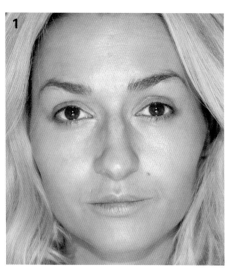

1. Quickly moisturize your face to create a smooth base, then apply a BB cream or a light foundation to even out the skin tone. Use your fingers – quicker than using a brush.

2. Cream eyeshadows are great for saving time as they are quicker to blend than powder shadows. Using the tip of your ring finger, apply a light brown cream eyeshadow over the entire eyelid, blend the edges into the skin, then brush on a layer of light brown or sheer powder to set.

3. Curl your lashes. This will open your eyes more and allow you to get away with skipping eyeliner, which can take time to apply. Add a quick sweep of mascara.

Pro's tip

There are some great contouring and highlighting duos on the market, starting with Sleek at the cheaper end and finishing with Tom Ford at the top end. They are easy to use and will save you time and space in your makeup bag.

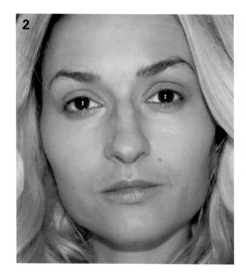

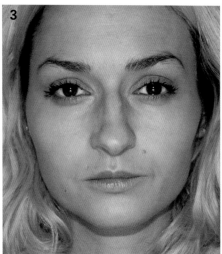

4. Apply a bit of blusher along the cheekbones or bronzer below them, just to define the contours of your face.

5. Use a tinted lip gloss on the lips. It's quicker to apply than lipstick and you don't need to spend time perfecting the outline.

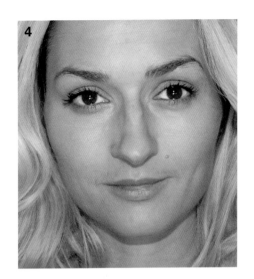

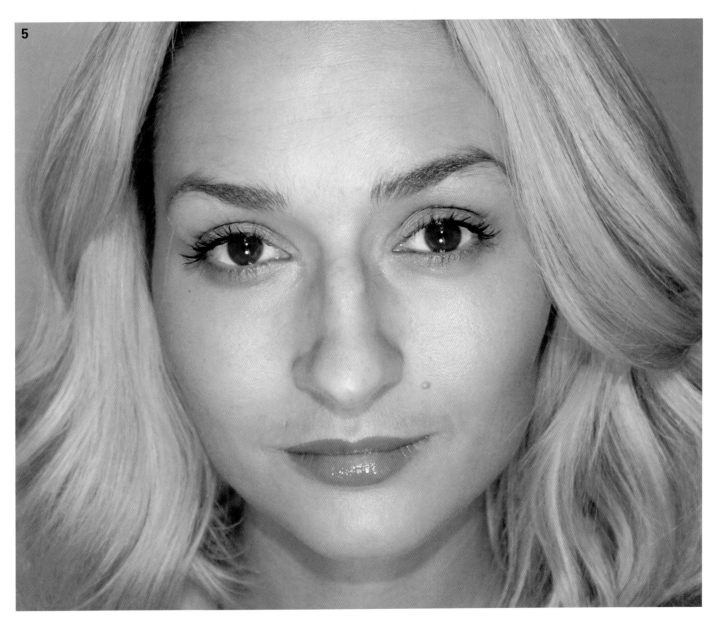

Anti-ageing makeup tips

As your face ages, its shape, skin tone and features can all change dramatically and the makeup routine that's served you well all your life may not do so any more. With a few simple tricks, you can update your look and enhance the areas of your face that need a boost.

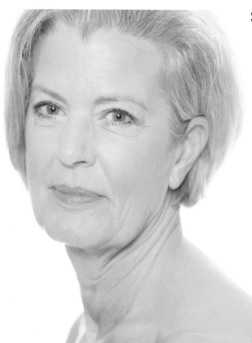

SKIN

Always moisturize before applying your base to plump up the skin and temporarily smooth out those lines.

Your skin may be showing some pigmentation. While the temptation is to go heavy on the concealer and foundation, an overly made-up look can really age the face. Focus concealer only on the areas of really uneven tone and leave the rest of your skin as natural as you can get away with.

Skin loses moisture with age, so if you've always used powder formulas, switch to cream or liquid foundation and blush to avoid a chalky finish. Powders also settle into lines, emphasizing rather than hiding them.

Using a primer will also help to smooth out lines.

Seek out illuminating foundations or BB creams that will reflect the light, giving the illusion of glowing, youthful skin.

If you want to use a powder to set your foundation, make it a loose, translucent one.

Use shadowing to hide sagging by dusting a light touch of matt bronzer along the neck and jaw line.

EYES

To avoid emphasizing fine lines, steer clear of shimmer, glitter and metallic eyeshadows.

Very pale matt colours will also age you, so look for soft, well-pigmented matts in natural tones such as taupes, plums and muted olive.

Contouring around the eye socket becomes less defined as the lids begin to droop. To replace some depth, open your eye really wide and use a neutral colour on an eyeshadow brush to trace along the socket line where the eyelid meets the bone, gently blending.

LASHES

The lashline will lose colour as lashes get sparser; a good trick is to dot a bit of eyeliner pencil very low between the lashes to give the illusion of thickness at the roots.

Curling the lashes also helps to open up the eye and give a lift to heavy lids. Mascara is your best friend as you age and the one product you should never leave out; look for volumizing formulas.

Strip lashes are too much, but for an evening look try out individual lash inserts or corner lashes. They can be tricky to handle at first, but once you have mastered the technique you'll find they give a really natural-looking fullness.

BROWS

As you age, the brows get thinner and lose shape, especially if you overplucked them when younger. Growth serums are great for helping regain some natural thickness.

You can cheat fuller brows. If you have a few patchy areas, try a brow powder a shade lighter than your natural brow to fill in gaps without a heavy finish.

If you have lost shape completely, a very sharp brow pencil can be used to gently sketch in small strokes that mimic natural hairs. Never draw on block colour, and keep it slightly lighter than your brow or hair colour.

You can also get semi-permanent brow pens with a super-fine tip that give a similar effect and last really well.

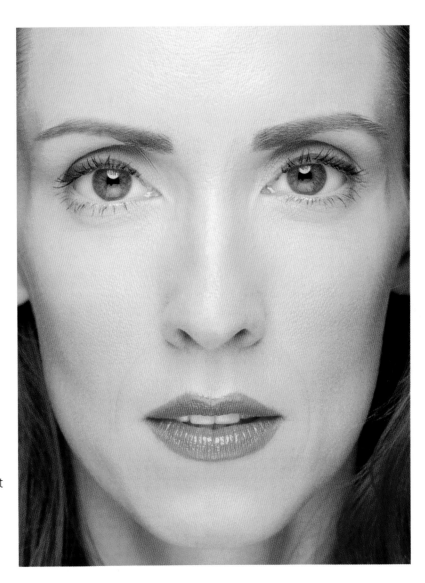

LIPS

As you get older the lips can become thinner, lose fullness and lack definition around the border. Warm, peachy shades are the most flattering on lips and cheeks. Avoid pale pinks and very dark colours.

Use a lip liner and gently buff on colour. Don't create a harsh line. Use the liner on the whole lip and gently around the edge, filling out any uneven areas to give definition and prevent colour from bleeding.

Follow with lipstick and, to finish, add a light slick of gloss to create the illusion of volume.

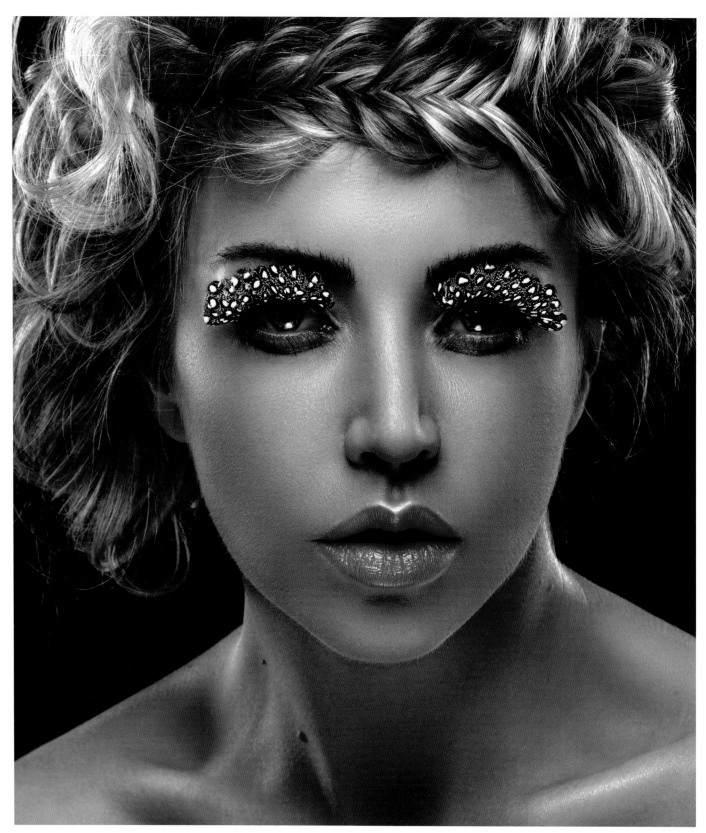

A goddess-inspired, high-impact look styled by pro MUA Anne Bowcock

Chapter Six

High Impact

Some occasions call for all-out glamour and a polished perfection that will carry you through from day to night. Whether it's the party of the year, an ultra-glam red carpet event, a school prom or even your wedding day, the right makeup will make sure you leave a lasting impression – and look fantastic in the high-def photos.

Go bold with sultry, smoky eyes or stand out with pops of neon colour to turn heads on a night out. Alternatively, keep occasion makeup pared back for daytime, and make an impact through perfectly flawless and luminous skin and groomed brows, paired with the prettiest soft blush and lip colour to suit your skin tone.

Remember, you can still create a big impression without making too much effort. There are plenty of time-savers on the market to see you through the day and all night long. Smudge on black cream shadow for a super-swift smoky eye or swap that perfect red lip for a high-colour gloss when you need glamour on the go. Experiment with some techniques and tips from the professionals to help you out of a makeup rut, and get creative with some of these looks to kill.

Day to night

Juggling work, family and a social life means it's hard for most women to find the time to create a whole new makeup look for that after work date or dinner with friends. By keeping daytime makeup light but long-wearing, you can avoid that caked-on layered look while creating a base to build on later and saving valuable time before a night out.

SASCHA JACKSON'S STEP-BY-STEP GUIDE TO A DAY-TO-NIGHT LOOK

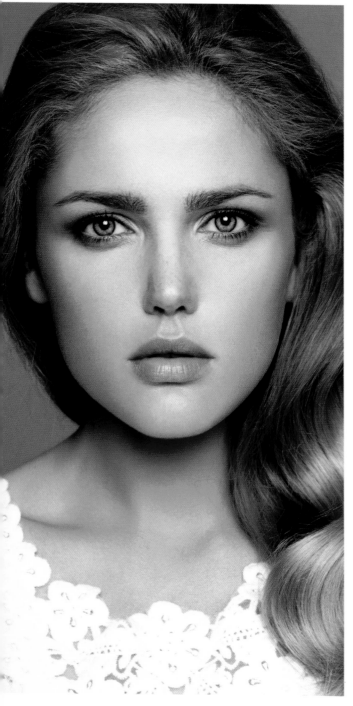

Day

1. Apply a long-lasting foundation because your base is the last thing you want to be worrying about before you head out. I love Stila's Stay All Day foundations because they are hydrating, leaving skin fresh and soft, plus they have a matching concealer in the lid for touch ups.

2. On the eyes, start your day with a matt, defined look by using a nude shadow over the lid and a natural brown or grey to contour in the socket. This will be easy to build on later when you want to add more. Then use a pencil eyeliner just to define the lashline.

3. If you want to load up on the mascara for the evening then try using just a clear mascara during the day. This way, when you apply black mascara later, you avoid clumping and those spider-leg lashes.

4. Add a pop of colour to the cheeks using a cream blush to keep the skin looking fresh.

PROFILE
SASCHA JACKSON

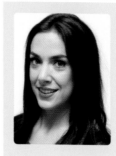

Sascha Jackson worked for one of the top French makeup houses before joining Stila in 2013, quickly becoming a pro-artist for the brand. She has since been appointed brand ambassador and now represents Stila on television and at media events.

Night

1. Begin the transition by adding a darker, matt shadow in the socket of the eye over the look you created in the morning. This will add drama and depth to your eyes.

2. Now use a shimmer pigment over the lid to transform the look into a more glamorous evening effect. I'd suggest using Stila Magnificent Metals or a similar metallic loose powder eyeshadow for this. Use a brush to press it gently over your existing shadow.

3. Using the same pencil eyeliner you applied in the morning, add a bolder line across the lashline and smudge it to create a soft, sultry finish.

4. Add bronzer in the natural contours of your cheeks to enhance the shape of your face, then apply more of the blush along your cheekbones.

5. Slick a dark, bold gloss on top of your daytime lip for a strong look.

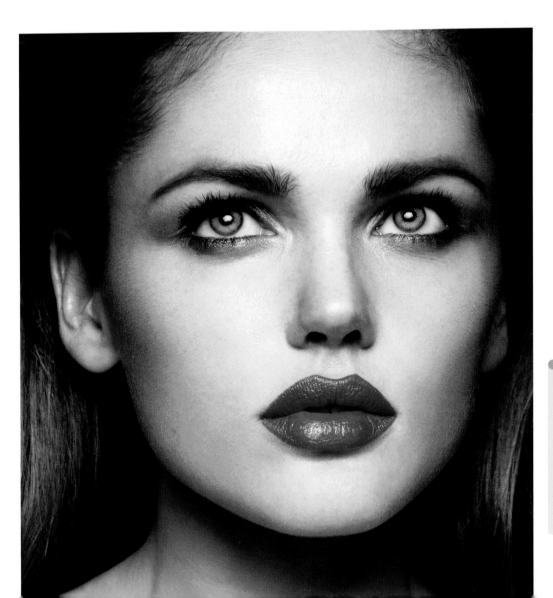

Pro's tip

If you can't bear the thought of a day without your trusty black mascara, then apply one light layer in the morning so you can still build on it later.

Red carpet glamour

A red-carpet-ready evening look means sultry eyes, glossy lips and plenty of illuminators to catch the light from those paparazzi flashlights. But for a hi-def photo finish, pro MUA Sascha Jackson says the real secret is in the skin.

On the red carpet, complexions always look naturally flawless. To achieve this without using a lot of foundation, Sascha suggests using a BB cream with illuminating pigments and mixing it in with your normal foundation before applying. 'The key is to mix about one part BB cream to three parts foundation,' she says. 'The result is amazing; you get skin that looks like a flawless, naturally glowing version of your own skin. I wouldn't send anyone down the red carpet without it.'

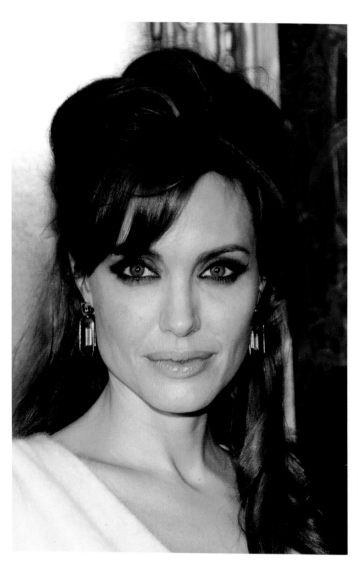
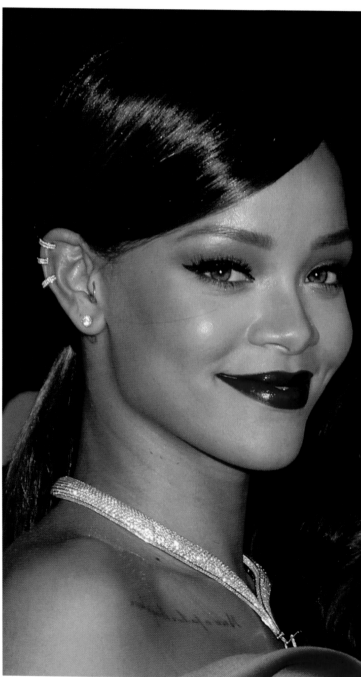

Celebrity red carpet glamour makeup (left to right): Angelina Jolie, Rhianna, Jennifer Lawrence, Lupita Nyong'o

SASCHA JACKSON'S STEP-BY-STEP GUIDE TO RED CARPET GLAMOUR

1. Mix your foundation and illuminating BB base, then apply it with a flat-top foundation brush and buff into the skin with a circular motion.

2. Use a cream-textured product in a darker shade than your skin tone to contour your face below the cheekbones, at the sides of the nose and below the jaw.

3. Highlight the high points of the face, nose and cheekbones. Use a glimmery, wet-look product with pearlescent tones that will capture the light and make your cheekbones pop.

4. Apply a dark gel liner all over the lid – then buff it out. This will give a quick base for that sultry, smoky eye. Pat a metallic pigment shadow on to the lid and blend away, leaving the edges soft and faded. This gives such a sexy finish and is quick to do. As the base is gel liner, you get no drop down from a shadow so there's no need to worry about panda eyes.

5. As the focus is on the eyes, keep lips neutral. Go for a lip gloss shade slightly warmer than your skin tone. The light-reflecting particles in a gloss give the illusion of a fuller lip. Use a neutral lipliner on the Cupid's bow and below the centre of the bottom lip. This will ensure your pout is perfectly defined and give your lips a boost.

Pro's tips

For red carpet makeup, I prefer not to overdo it with blush. Keep the face simple and structured with just contouring and highlighting, and let your eyes be the focus.

*

Before applying makeup, I love using moisturizing sheet face masks such as MaskerAide's Pre Party Prep mask to energize, hydrate and prime the skin. They make your makeup easier to apply and longer lasting.

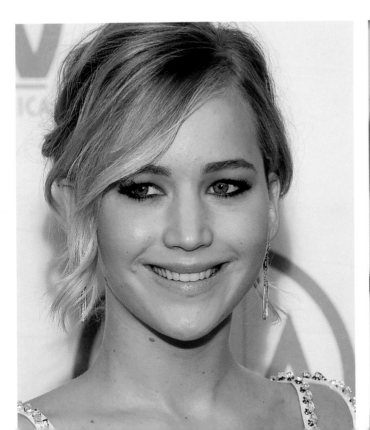

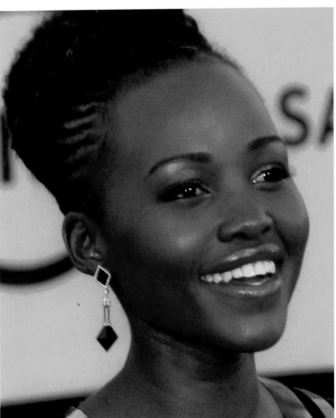

Prom makeup

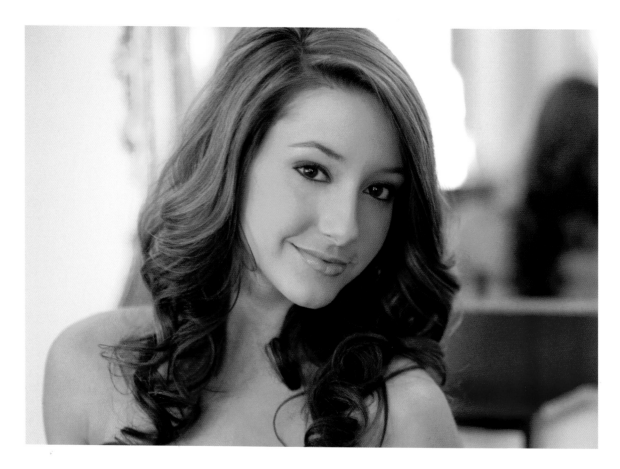

Prom makeup is one of the services most requested of a jobbing makeup artist. Any teenage girl or mum will value the following advice on how to perfect a party look that gives plenty of sparkle without too much of a heavy, grown-up finish. Many girls will choose a sparkly dress for a prom, so try a fresh, pretty look with plenty of shimmer to complement your standout dress without overpowering it. For extra glamour, consider going for a professional spray tan or try a home-use instant tan mousse which can be applied on the day and will easily wash off if there are any streaks.

Pro's tip

Use foundation with full coverage and long wear so it will stay put even when you're perspiring on the dance floor.

PROFILE
KIRSTIE BOWER

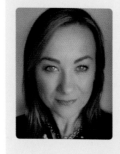

Kirstie Bower worked as an in-house trainer for several makeup companies before setting up her own business doing wedding and special occasion makeup. After eight years she joined Gerrard International to help launch the Mii makeup range, for which she is now area manager, training MUAs to use the products.

KIRSTIE BOWER'S STEP-BY-STEP GUIDE TO THE PROM LOOK

1. Apply a primer to ensure that the look will stay fresh all night.

2. Colour match the foundation to the jawline and neck. Many girls go for a spray tan before the prom and this will vastly alter the skin tone, so bear this in mind.

3. Use a green-toned concealer where needed, to neutralize any redness before applying the base, then apply the foundation using a foundation brush. Try a mineral powder foundation such as Mii Mineral Irresistible Face Base as this is great for teenage skins which might be oily or prone to acne.

4. Powder the whole face with a mineral setting powder using a large brush.

5. Using a contour palette and angled brush, contour under the cheekbones and jawline and around the crease of the eyelid, then add highlighter above the eyes.

6. Use a pretty pink shimmer mineral blush on the apples of the cheeks to give fullness. Apply this with a smaller, natural-hair brush.

A fresh, shimmery teenage prom look by Kirstie Bower

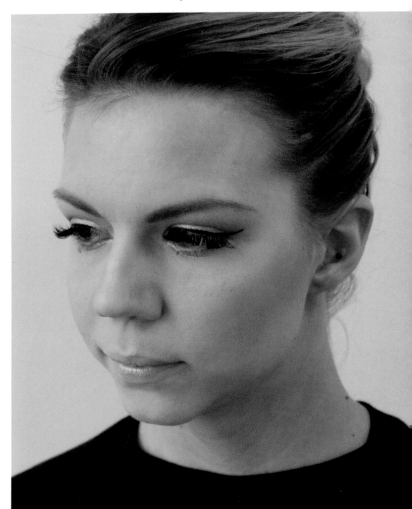

7. Choose a shimmer pressed eyeshadow in a light colour – I picked one with a hint of lilac metallic to complement the model's dark eye colour – and use a small, natural-hair eyeshadow brush to apply it over the top lid and around the inner corner of the eye, extending to slightly below the lower lid. Highlight under the browbone with a paler shimmer pressed shadow, then blend with a medium socket blender brush.

8. Use a liquid liner applied in a very fine line, close to the lashes and extended in a flick. Professional salon lash extensions (like the ones the model is wearing) are fantastic for a prom, but strip lashes could be applied instead after the liner. Then add black mascara to the bottom lashes.

9. Keep the brows nice and full, but define and extend them slightly using a dark brown defining pencil and waterproof brow shadow.

10. To finish the look, add a slick of baby pink shimmer gloss to the lips.

Party style

For a party or big night out, make the eyes sparkle with metallics, shimmers or glitters for a look that's sexy, but contemporary. Leave the smoky eye behind and use strong black as a definer only, via a crisp liner and thick lashes. Go bright with a pop of colour on the lips; try a matt finish to contrast with the shimmer of the eyes or add gloss for a full-on party shine.

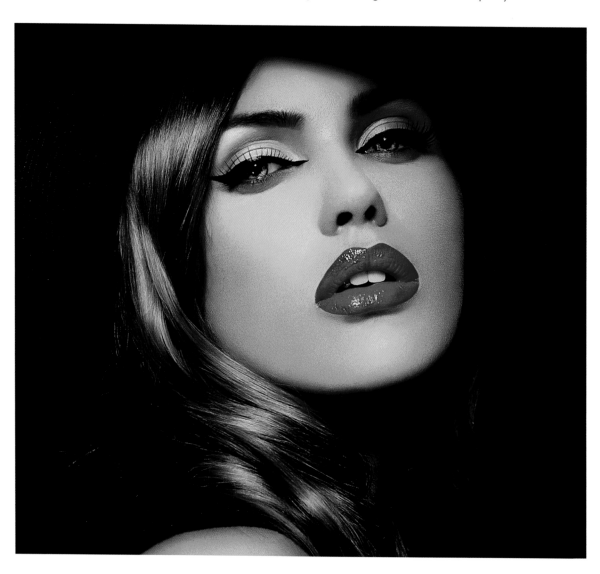

PROFILE
KELLIE LICORISH

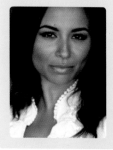

Kellie Licorish specializes in both traditional and airbrush makeup techniques and currently heads up the team for Mistair Airbrush makeup and Stage Line Professional HD makeup. Kellie has worked backstage on catwalk shows for London Fashion Week, Milan Fashion Week and Paris Haute Couture Week. She has also worked with celebrities, including Rita Ora and Eliza Doolittle.

KELLIE LICORISH'S STEP-BY-STEP GUIDE TO A PARTY LOOK

1. Cleanse, tone, moisturize and prime to hydrate and prep the skin for a long night ahead.

2. Using a makeup brush or sponge, apply a full-coverage cream base that will stay put as the night hots up. Stage Line Professional H-Definition Cover is good as it is made with silicone to correct uneven skin.

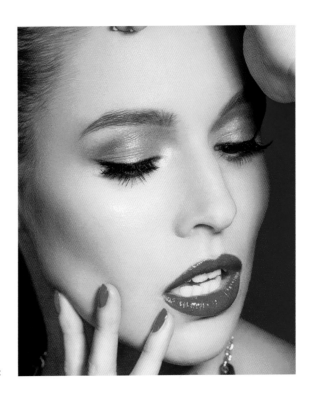

3. Every party look needs a hint of sparkle. Dust a chrome eyeshadow powder on the eyes, cheekbones and décolletage to give a luminous sheen.

4. Add a pop of colour with a liquid or cream blush applied to the apples of the cheeks in circular motions, lightly fading out to contour.

5. An eye primer is essential to stop makeup on the lids from creasing and becoming oily. Spread evenly, then add your metallic or glitter shadow. Use a powder formula to gradually build the colour in layers. Cover the lid and blend at the outer corner to the socket line.

6. Use a black eyeliner pen to accentuate the outer edges of the eyes and make the lashes stand out. Start at the outer edge and work in, making the line thinner so that it gradually fades into the lashline.

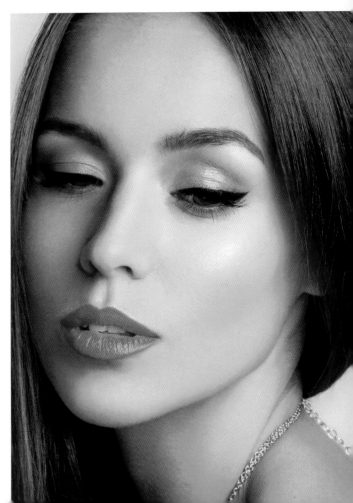

7. Add black mascara or, for more impact, apply false lashes to accentuate and open up the eyes.

8. For the perfect party pout, line and then colour in the lips using a lipliner to give a strong base. Use a lip brush to apply a bright lipstick in a colour that contrasts with your eye makeup without clashing. Add a lip gloss over your lipstick for super glossy lips that wow!

Glamour makeup

For party makeup, a lot of people want that full-on look with heavy eyes, statement lips and contoured cheeks, but you don't need to go all-out for your features to look great. When aiming for high impact, it's easy to overdo it.

For a look that's strong but still sophisticated, focus the heavy colour on either the eyes or the lips. Don't be heavy-handed with the bronzer or tan and remember to contour subtly. Full-coverage foundation will look flat and fake without contouring, but overdo the shading and you'll look stripy and strange.

As long as you keep the less-is-more mantra in mind, you'll be fine to grab the false lashes with confidence and go for glamour.

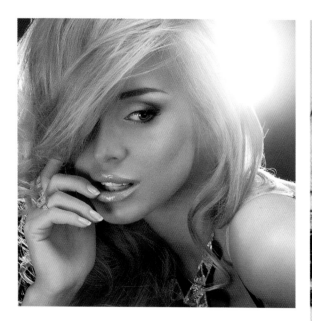

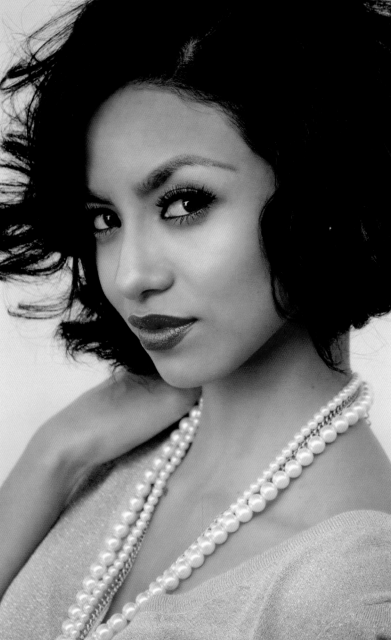

Pro's tip

If you look overdone, blend and blend some more. If your eyes are too dark or your contour too heavy, grab a clean brush and blend the product out using circular motions.

JEN HUNTER'S STEP-BY-STEP GUIDE TO GLAMOUR MAKEUP

1. Start on your eyes with a slight shimmer base that contrasts with your eye colour. Take it around the inner corner of the eye to catch the light and make your eyes open up and stand out.

2. Blend this out to a darker colour – black for full impact, dark brown for a softer finish. Blend these colours into each other using circular, controlled motions with your brush.

3. Pick a highlight that's not too glittery. A slight shimmer that is close to your skin tone works best. Use this to blend eyeshadow upwards from the crease to the browbone.

4. For added drama, line your eyes with a gel or liquid liner in dark brown or black. Take an angled brush and run this along your lashline on the top and bottom lids. For a more smoked-out look, take a thin brush and run this over the line you created; this will blend it out and soften the line.

5. False lashes add glamour, but make sure they're right for your eye shape. Before applying glue, measure the lashes up against your eye and cut at the outer end of the strip. After applying, run a coat of mascara through to blend your natural lashes with the false ones.

6. Move on to your foundation and ensure this matches your skin from your jawline to your neck.

7. Add contour to define the cheekbones. Look for a thin cream with a slight grey undertone to emulate shadow on your face and draw your cheekbones in. Add this under your cheekbones and jawline and around your hairline, then blend well.

8. Add highlight to the top points of your face, including down the centre of the nose, tops of cheeks, under the browbone and on your Cupid's bow. Finish with a slight dusting of blush to give the cheeks some warmth.

9. Using lipliner, draw on your lipline to ensure the colour stays all night. Cover the lips with your lipstick, then add a dot of gloss in the middle of the lips to make them pop.

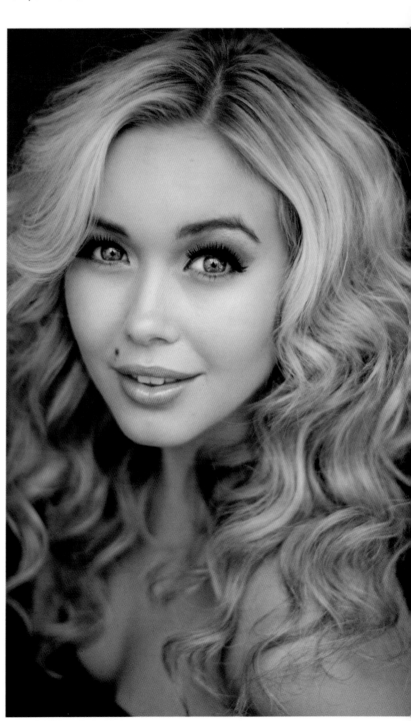

A high-glamour makeup look by Jen Hunter

Beautiful brides

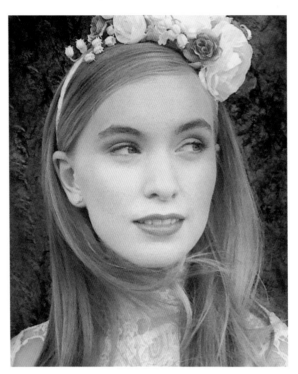

Whether you're preparing for the biggest day of your life or simply wanting to re-create that natural radiance all brides seem to emanate, bridal makeup techniques can give you a flawless finish with all-day wear.

Most women choose to enlist the help of a professional makeup artist on their wedding day, but you'll probably want to practise at home first to get a feel for the kind of look you'll want to discuss with your MUA. Meanwhile, if you decide to save some pennies and go it alone, there are loads of professional tricks you can use to create that dewy perfection all brides long for.

The English rose bridal makeup look by Alyn Waterman

CHOOSING THE LOOK

Classic and vintage makeup styles work well and stand the test of time when you look back at your photographs. If you're using a makeup artist for your wedding day, arrange a trial well in advance to discuss your colour choices and any themes you may have. Be clear about what you want and always check for any sensitivity or allergies to products they use.

Check your finished makeup in daylight to make sure you're happy with it. Above all, aim for a more enhanced, polished version of how you normally look – you want your groom to recognize you when you walk down the aisle!

PROFILE
ALYN WATERMAN

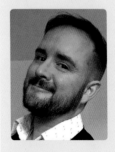

Makeup and hair artist Alyn Waterman is a firm favourite with award-winning actresses and celebrities. He has been the personal hair stylist and on-set makeup artist to Hollywood legend Dame Joan Collins for more than 10 years. With over 25 years' experience, Alyn has worked widely in television and on advertising campaigns for Avon, Schwarzkopf and Dermalogica.

The prep

A white dress can wash out your skin tone, so many brides go for a professional spray tan a couple of days before the wedding. Take your time finding the right person and again trial the formulation a few weeks in advance. If you top it up with body makeup on the day, remember to set it well with powder to avoid staining your dress.

Everyone aspires to a fresh, dewy look to the skin. To achieve this, use thin layers of makeup and don't overload your skin with too many products. Start with a good primer – Alyn recommends Dermalogica Skin Perfect Primer – then follow with a long-lasting concealer such as Joan Collins Timeless Beauty Fade to Perfect to cover dark circles. Choose an illuminating foundation such as Bourjois Healthy Mix, then set it with a loose powder that also offers a light sheen such as Le Maq Pro HD Powder.

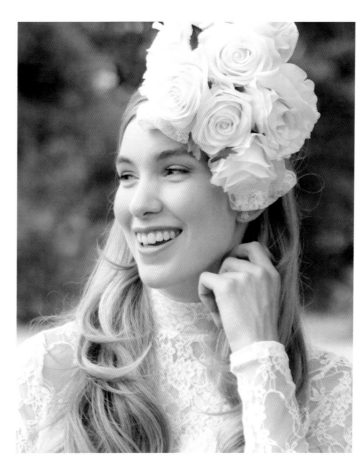

The eyes

Use waterproof products around your eyes so if you do shed a tear you won't shed your makeup with it. There are some great semi-permanent eyeliners available now, as well as long-lasting waterproof mascaras. For eye colour, prime the lids and choose cream shadows for longevity. MAC Pro Longwear Paint Pots last well.

The cheeks and lips

A pink or peachy colour is lovely on the apples of the cheeks. Stipple it on and blend it in for that flushed finish. Try Art Deco Blush 23 or Revlon Photoready Cream Blush. On the lips, use crayons rather than glossy lipsticks to give a soft colour. Lip stains are long-lasting, but make sure you apply a gloss on top to stop the lips feeling dry.

Finally, a setting spray is always a good option for all-day wear – try Skindinavia Bridal Makeup Finish.

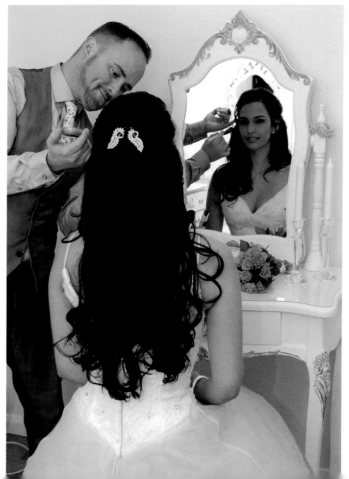

Top: makeup by Alyn Waterman

Right: Alyn Waterman at work

High-impact bridal

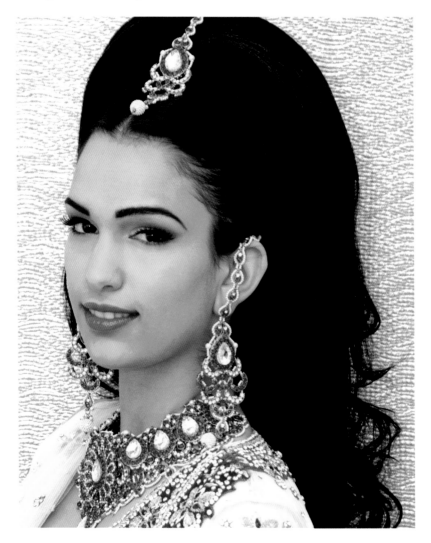

The subtle, classic look will always be a wedding day staple, but many modern brides want to make more of a statement. When all eyes – and camera lenses – are on you, it's sometimes worth considering taking the natural look up a gear for classic glamour that's high-impact yet never trashy.

ALYN WATERMAN'S STEP-BY-STEP GUIDE TO HIGH-IMPACT BRIDAL

1. Prep and prime skin thoroughly before makeup application to ensure that your makeup lasts all day. Use foundation first, then concealer; build up the foundation from the centre panel of the face, sweeping out towards the hairline in thin layers. Use a cheek highlighter to create a dewy finish. Set the base with a mineral veil powder.

2. Add a light bronzer to warm the skin tone. I also used a darker bronzer below the cheekbones to contour the face.

3. Define the eyebrows with brow powder and an angled brush, using short feathery strokes to build up the shape.

4. Shade your eyes using three tones of light, medium and dark eyeshadow. With a foam applicator, highlight the inner corner and browbone with a light shade. Choose a medium-warm colour to contour the socket, then add a deep shade on the outer lid and into the socket. Blend all of these using a clean, soft blending brush.

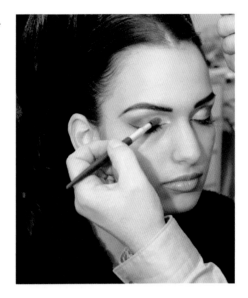

5. Add a black eyeshadow along the top and bottom lashlines for a smoky effect, then apply waterproof mascara.

6. Add false lashes along the top lashline, then use a black liquid liner to create extra depth between the lid and the lash.

7. Use a soft rose blush on the cheeks. I also brushed a little over the eyes to bring all the makeup colours together.

8. Apply base and powder over the lips, then use a red lipliner to define the shape and fill in the lips completely to create a base. Powder lightly, then apply a soft red lipstick using a lip brush. These steps will help your lipstick last longer.

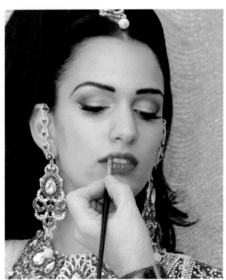

9. Finish with a light mist of makeup fixing spray to ensure your look lasts all day and throughout the evening's party.

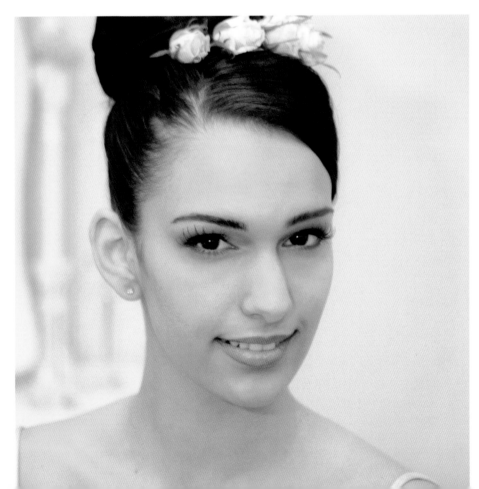

All bridal makeup by Alyn Waterman

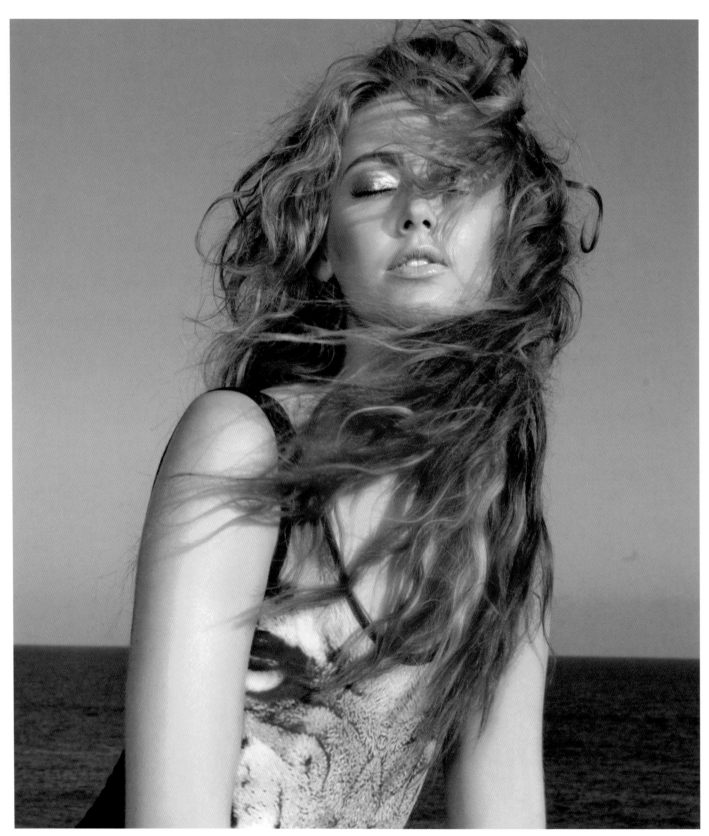

A metallic eye look from a fashion editorial shoot by Abbi-Rose Crook

Chapter Seven

Fashion Forward

Just as couture fashion filters through to more wearable high-street looks, makeup innovation often makes its first appearance on the catwalk. Every season, makeup artists look to the runways of Milan, London, Paris and New York for the cosmetic colours and techniques that will shape new trends.

Professional makeup artists working backstage at the fashion weeks take their cue from the fashion designers they are working with, coming up with looks to complement the label's next season collection. While some designers want the makeup pared back so as not to overshadow the clothes, others give the artists free rein to make the face as crazily creative as the couture. Trends such as graphic liner, gold leaf and the matt orange lip all made their debut on the catwalk, quickly working their way into every makeup artist's box of tricks, along with more subtle staples such as perfect dewy skin and deep berry lips.

Campaign and editorial shoots are also incubators for bold, experimental looks, especially with an edgy celeb as the star. Think Kate Moss kicking off grunge-chic on the cover of *Vogue*, or Katy Perry popularizing 50s chic in her ghd campaign.

But the real skill lies in making these looks wearable for the everyday woman who isn't blessed with a five-hour session in hair and makeup before she sets off for work. The makeup artists responsible for creating the magic behind the catwalk and in front of the lens have plenty of tips for re-creating standout looks, achieving the perfect high-definition finish and making makeup last all day long. They also share their tips and tricks for fast fashion fixes, such as adhesive liners and accessories that channel catwalk trends with a minimum of fuss.

Dewy skin

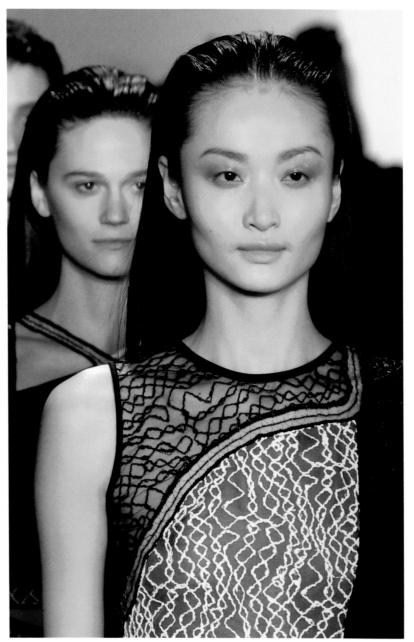

If there's one look that defines fashion and editorial makeup, it's dewy skin. When catwalk models hit the runway, the designer wants their skin to look fresh and glowing. Whether it's complemented with subtle eyes and lips or used as a base for pop colour, skin has to look natural.

Meanwhile, the high-def finish of photoshoots makes the powdery or chalky finish a no-no. 'At all the catwalk shows I've done, the designers want the girls to look glowing and healthy, and in editorial shoots they often won't let you use powder, as it shows up in the photos and looks unnatural. The skin needs to look like skin,' says makeup artist Louise Dartford, who has worked on shoots for the likes of *Elle* and *Grazia* magazines.

Early starts, late nights and back-to-back shows mean that many young models don't have great skin, but you'd never know it once the professional makeup artists have finished with them. Heavy cover-ups may hide blemishes, but they also cover all the good skin. By focusing your coverage only on the blemishes and leaving the rest of the skin as natural as possible, you can re-create a look that's flawless, not fake.

PROFILE
LOUISE DARTFORD

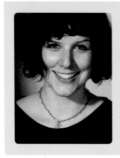

Louise Dartford has worked on fashion campaigns for All Saints, ASOS and Liberty, and shows for Alchemy and Zandra Rhodes. Her celebrity music clients have included Dizzee Rascal and Tinchy Stryder and she's done editorial work for *InStyle*, *Esquire* and *Elle*, among others. Lou's passion is organic and natural beauty.

Pro's tip

Dewy skin looks great with subtle eyes (groomed brows and a slick of black mascara for definition), but it's also great with a heavier smoky eye.

LOUISE DARTFORD'S STEP-BY-STEP GUIDE TO DEWY SKIN

1. Apply a very light foundation or a tinted moisturizer all over as a base. A lot of people reach for a heavy foundation to cover everything up and get a completely uniform finish, but that will always look fake.

2. Use a good concealer to paint out blemishes. I always use a dry rather than cream textured concealer, and a small, fine brush. Target individual blemishes rather than painting the whole face.

3. Use gentle strokes to cover the blemish, working outwards from the centre and blending. Then dab it with your finger and repeat the process two or three times.

4. You'll now have two to three fine layers, which will last better and look far more natural than one thick layer. Repeat the process for all blemishes you want to cover.

5. Continue the dewiness with a light application of blusher. Use a cream not a powder brush and apply along the cheekbones, blending up and out. A lot of people go wrong with blusher by applying it to the apples of the cheeks when smiling and blending downwards. This drags the whole face down and draws attention to the nose area and down, rather than the eyes.

6. Set the look with a dusting of very finely milled powder. RMK and Illamasqua do great ones.

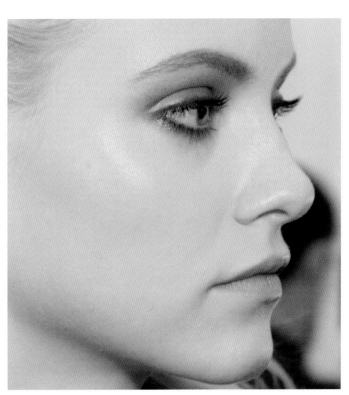
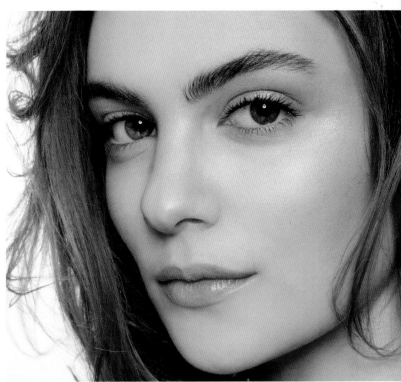

The bleached brow

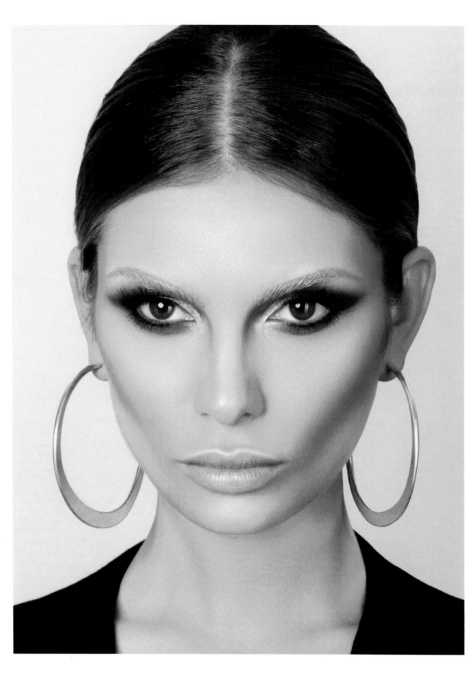

The bleached brow or 'no brow' effect has been a hot look on the catwalks – a reaction to the heavily defined or brushed-up brows that have dominated in recent years. The bleached brow look has a 90s revival vibe and turns the face into a blank canvas. Most models who walk the runway with this look will have their brow colour stripped with a facial hair bleach such as Jolen, then tinted back after the show. However, on photo shoots, MUAs usually can't do anything permanent or semi-permanent to the model because their agency contracts don't allow it. So some use concealer to fake the bleached look, which is a great cheat you can use to try out the effect at home.

This look works best on women with a strong bone structure. It doesn't suit everyone because you are effectively taking a feature away from the face, so it will dramatically change your appearance. However, as you are only using concealer, if you don't like it you can wash it straight off. It is best suited to those with pale skin and looks the most dramatic when paired with a heavy, smoky eye.

PROFILE
ABBI-ROSE CROOK

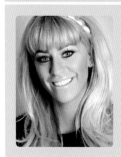

Abbi-Rose Crook works as a makeup artist across fashion, celebrity, beauty, editorial and TV. Her work has taken her around the world with established photographers, celebrities and corporate clients. She won the Professional Beauty Award for Makeup Specialist of the Year in 2012. Abbi-Rose has a background in beauty therapy, so is also adept at creating beautiful skin and nails.

ABBI-ROSE CROOK'S STEP-BY-STEP GUIDE TO THE BLEACHED BROW LOOK

1. Use tweezers to shape the brow, because the outline will still show, even under concealer.

2. Using clear mascara, brush the hairs upwards. This will give a sticky base for the concealer to cling to.

3. Choose a fairly pale concealer. I usually use a peachy, off-white shade, but in general it should be lighter than you'd use on the rest of your face. The colour you use to cover dark undereye circles should work well.

4. Use a disposable mascara spoolie to apply the concealer, brushing the brows downwards and twisting the wand as you go so you cover the whole hair, then brush upwards into a smooth shape.

5. Blend any concealer on your face into your foundation using a concealer or foundation blending brush.

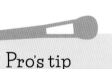

Pro's tip

If you find clear mascara too sticky, try starting with a concealer pencil. Its waxy formula will help coat the hairs evenly.

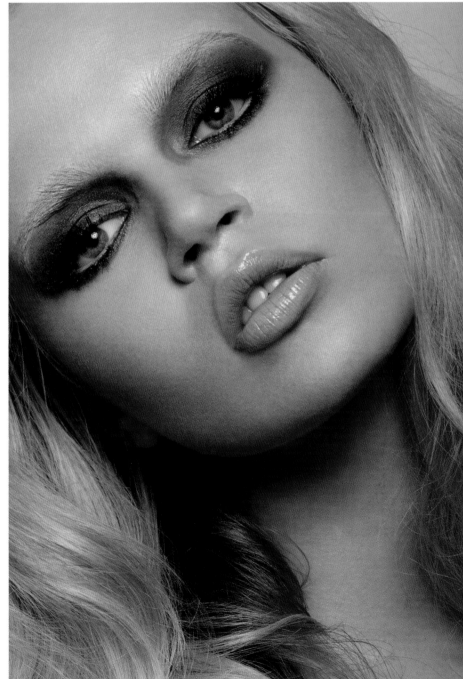

A bleached-effect brow created using concealer by Abbi-Rose Crook

The neon matt lip

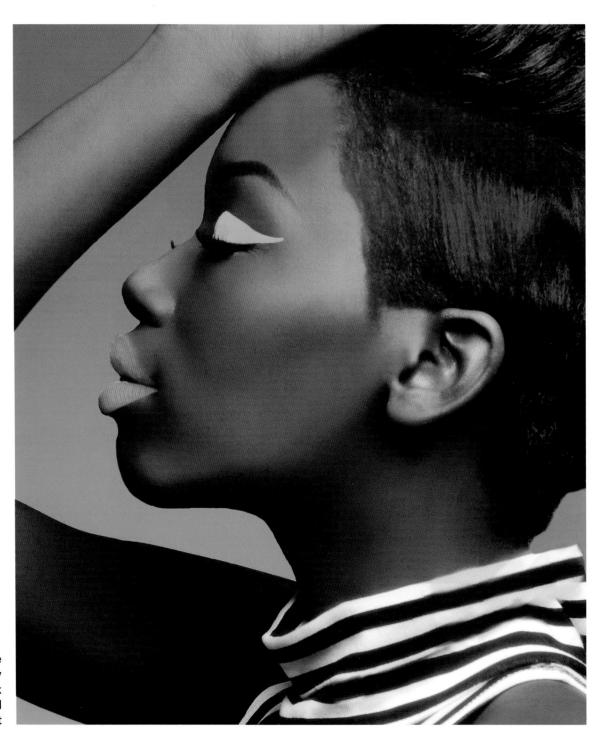

An extreme use of matt neons by Abbi-Rose Crook for an editorial shoot

Bold pop colours immediately make the lips a statement feature and are used time after time in editorial shoots to add instant edge. Bright lipstick is the quickest way to transform a look and going matt makes bright colours much easier to wear. Matts are longer lasting than gloss formulas. This look is better suited to younger women, as matt colours can be ageing. A gloss finish adds vitality to the lips and creates the illusion of fullness, whereas matt colours can flatten the area and be quite drying. But, with the right application, a pop of matt colour in a bright or even a neon shade looks confident and on trend, ensuring that all eyes are on you.

ABBI-ROSE CROOK'S GUIDE TO PERFECTING THE BRIGHT MATT LIP

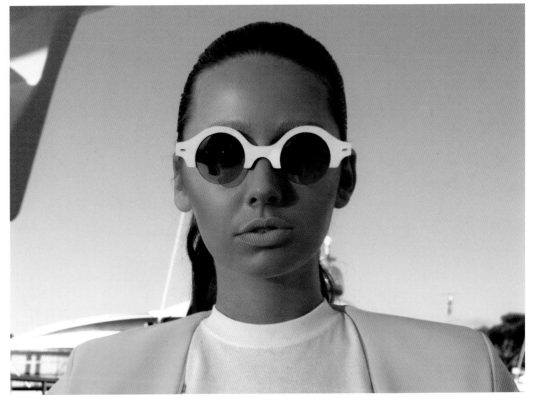

Bright matt lips stand out against flawless skin on an editorial look by Abbi-Rose Crook

1. Exfoliate the lips first, as a matt finish will magnify any dryness or flakiness there.

2. Moisturize to give a smooth base, but use a non-oily balm so there's no slip when you apply the colour.

3. Apply concealer to the whole lip area. This is a trick used by makeup artists because it creates a blank canvas. If you've ever bought a lipstick and been disappointed that it looks completely different when you apply it, it's because the natural pink of your lips is showing through.

4. Use a lip brush to apply the lipstick so that you get even coverage. If you apply straight from the bullet, the pressure will leave you with uneven product.

5. Use concealer, applied with a small synthetic brush, to neaten around the edges.

6. Finish with a lipliner to give a really crisp line, as both the brightness and the matt texture will cause any unevenness to show up.

7. Try adding a neon powder to finish. Use a finger to pat it into the lipstick, over the fuller part of the lip. This gives a 3D edge and makes lips appear more voluminous.

Pro's tip

When going neon on the lips, keep the rest of the makeup simple and neutral so the lips become the focal point, like a statement pair of shoes. Foundation should be luminescent, never matt, as the latter can look cakey against a bright matt lip.

The rock chick look

Rock and grunge makeup influences lend a timeless edginess to any look and are never off the catwalk for more than a season or two. Just as fashion designers team black leather with feminine chiffons to create a juxtaposition of textures, makeup artists will often pair glossy black eyeshadows with soft, dewy skin and nude lips, or deep burgundy lips with a natural eye. This creates an edgy look, but stops short of slipping into goth territory. If you want a fast but high-impact rock look, mastering a cream eyeshadow in black will give you a fantastically versatile base to experiment with.

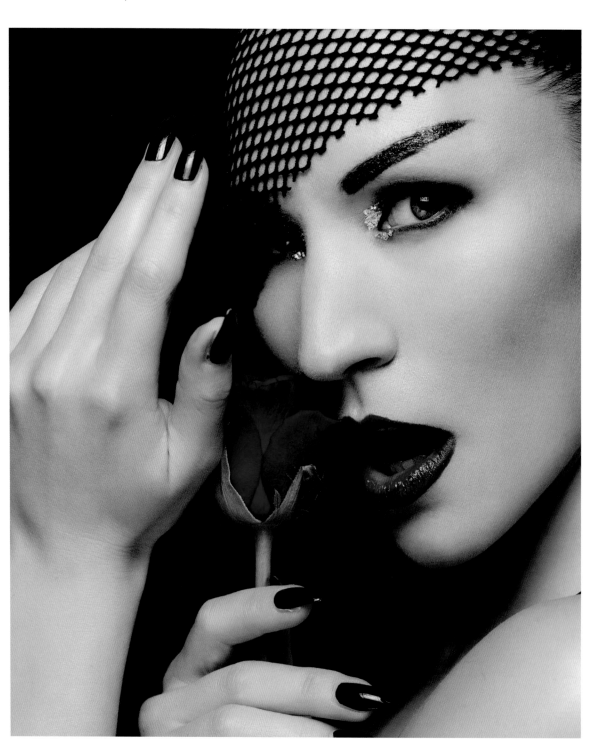

A vampy look created by pro MUA Pamela Moss

JO COLETTA'S STEP-BY-STEP GUIDE TO A WEARABLE ROCK CHICK LOOK

1. After prepping the skin and applying foundation and concealer, start with the eyes.

2. Apply a black cream eyeshadow over the lid and up to the browbone, then run the product under the lower lashline. MAC Pro Longwear Paint Pot in Blackground is a great choice for this. Then use a blending brush to soften the edges or blend outwards to create a winged effect.

3. To intensify, use a black kohl pencil to line the ring of the eye, including the inner waterline, and blend with a smaller brush. Add black mascara to the bottom and top lashes.

4. For a party look, you could add some silver or black glitter or pigment on top of the lid at this stage. For an editorial or catwalk finish, try adding a touch of clear lip gloss to the centre of the eyelids for a wet-look eye. This would be applied right at the last minute on a photo shoot or before a show, as it can cause the eye makeup to crease.

5. I lightened the model's brows with concealer for this shoot (above), but for a more wearable evening look just brush the brows up and, if necessary, fill them in slightly with brow pencil and set with a brow gel.

6. Slightly contour the cheeks, then set the look with a matt powder.

7. Use either a nude matt lipstick or gloss. To make the model's lips look extra pale, I brushed the excess foundation from my brush over them.

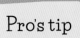

Pro's tip

If you want something more natural than black makeup, try the look using a bronze cream shadow and brown kohl pencil.

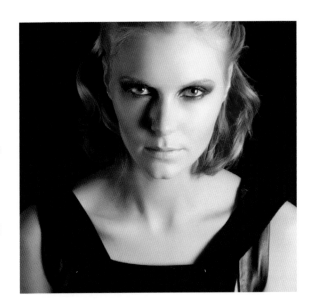

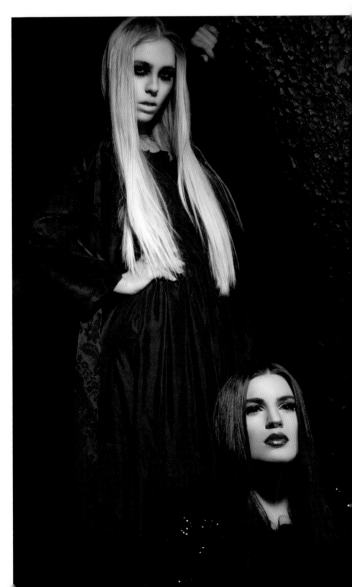

Top: a dark makeup look by Jo Coletta

Right: some dark, gothic looks created by MUA Abbi-Rose Crook

Fun fashion — embellishment

Adhesive embellishments have only really come into focus in the last decade as artists begin to push the boundaries on the catwalk and in editorial shoots. They were pioneered by fashion MUA Pat McGrath, then adopted by celebrities and performers such as Lady Gaga and Jessie J, looking to take makeup to the next level. In recent years companies such as Face Lace and Eye Rock have taken adhesive makeup more mainstream with elaborate graphic eyeliner styles. Meanwhile, the gold leaf effects seen on the catwalks at Fendi and Chanel have been translated by MAC and are also available as adhesive tattoos.

Face accessories are a step up from textures such as metallic shadows or glitter designs and can give a standout look for a party or a festival where you want to be the centre of attention.

Some accessories are self-adhesive and will come with application instructions. Others work like the fake tattoos for kids and involve applying water to the reverse, holding down the paper, then peeling off the backing to reveal the foil.

Embellishment with gold leaf tattoos done by Abbi-Rose Crook for a shoot for *Professional Beauty* magazine

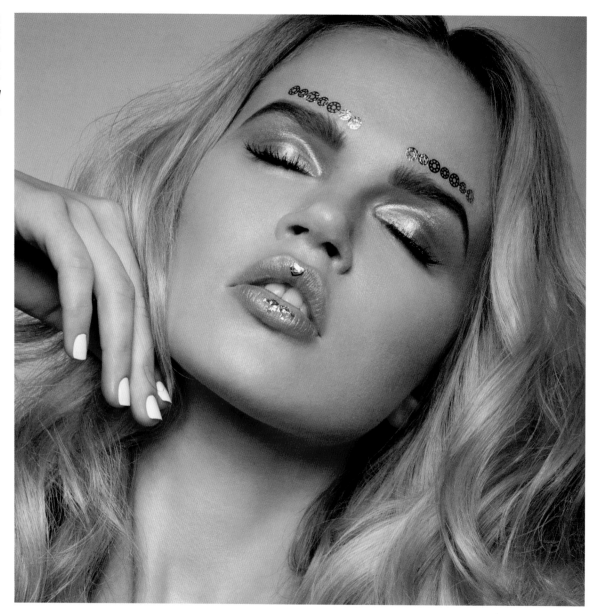

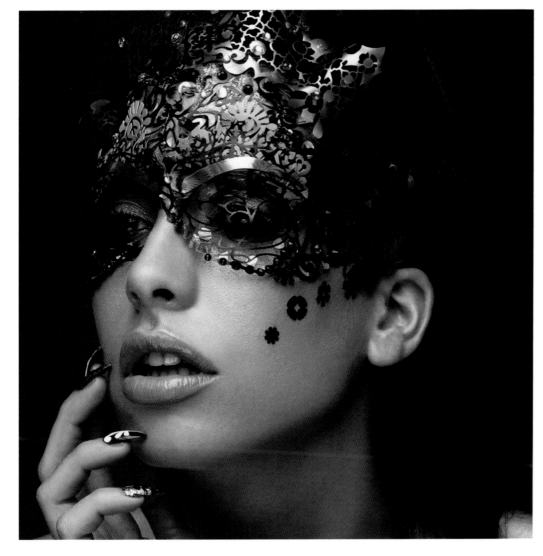

A fun fashion look styled for an editorial shoot by Abbi-Rose Crook, using Face Lace adhesive accessories

ABBI-ROSE CROOK'S PRO TIPS FOR MAKEUP EMBELLISHMENT

1. The picture on the facing page was done for a shoot so I went heavy on the gold, pairing a metallic eye with gold foil tattoos on the lips and above the brows.

2. For a more wearable look, for a party or a festival, less is more. Let either the eyes or the lips do the talking and keep the rest of the face neutral. So if you're applying lace-effect adhesives around the eyes, keep the lips plain or, for foil effect lips, go low key on the eyes.

3. Always start with very clean, dry skin to get the longest-lasting effect. Don't apply over cream or powder.

4. With black lace-effect adhesives, choose one key piece and keep colour to a minimum elsewhere on the face. Try pairing with a liquid liner flick and soft pink lip for a sophisticated look.

Makeup that lasts all day

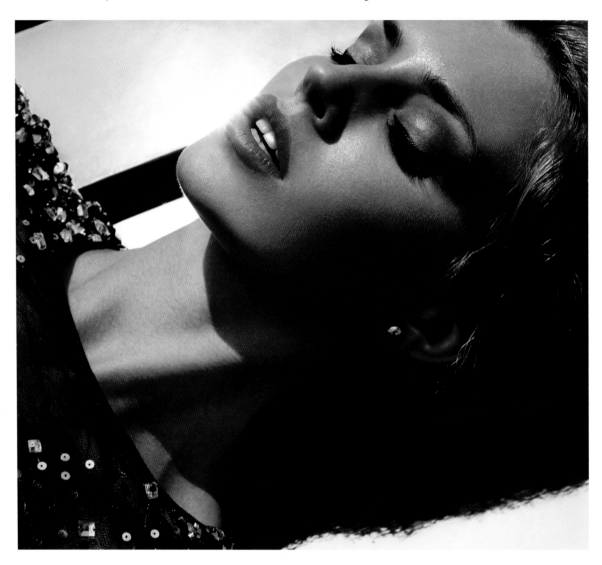

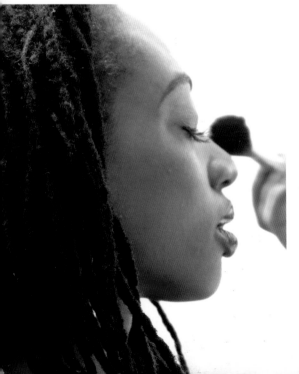

When working on editorial or video shoots, makeup artists have to keep their colour in place all day; they can't be buzzing around celebs mid-shot to touch up the base. Fortunately, there's a raft of tricks the pros can use to keep makeup looking fresh.

Your skin type will play a big role in how long your makeup lasts. Foundation seems to slide off oily skin whereas it will clump and flake on drier skins. But the good news is that there are products you can use both before and after applying makeup to balance and correct any skin flaws and keep your makeup put. There are also some great long-lasting products that stay strong for hours on end.

The most important trick to keeping makeup in place all day long, though, is layering. Celebrity makeup artist Aimee Adams suggests using a cream version of each product as a base, then layering it with a powder. She does this when applying foundation, eyeshadow and blusher, using very fine layers and setting them in between to create lasting hold without a thick, cakey finish.

AIMEE ADAMS'S STEP-BY-STEP GUIDE TO 24-HOUR MAKEUP

1. Preparation is the most important factor in keeping makeup in place. If you're using an exfoliator and a mask weekly, your skin should be in good shape. But if there's any flakiness, exfoliate and moisturize well before applying your base to make sure you start with smooth, dry skin.

2. Primer is the glue that holds your makeup to the skin, so start with a fine layer of wet primer then quickly apply your liquid foundation before it dries so that the layers set together. You could even try squeezing a little primer into your base before applying, so they work together.

3. Once you've applied your cream or liquid foundation, set it with a fine layer of loose translucent powder such as Corn Silk Powder.

4. Follow this with a loose powder foundation to set the colour, blending carefully.

5. Repeat this process for the cheeks and eyes, applying a cream colour first before a dusting of translucent powder, then a powder colour. Do your shading and blending over the powder layer.

6. For eyes, look out for 24-hour gel liners and waterproof mascaras. For brows, choose a kit that pairs a brow powder with a setting wax or gel to keep the powder in place.

Pro's tip

If your skin is oily or you are in a warm environment, use blotting papers to soak up any grease or sweat. They are great for keeping makeup perfect without adding more layers.

7. For lips, start with a lip stain, then layer it with pencil, powder and lipstick, blotting then reapplying the lipstick with a brush.

8. Set the whole face with another dusting of translucent powder.

9. You can make the look last even longer with a setting spray. Urban Decay do some good ones. But be careful with sprays, as they often contain alcohol and can be drying.

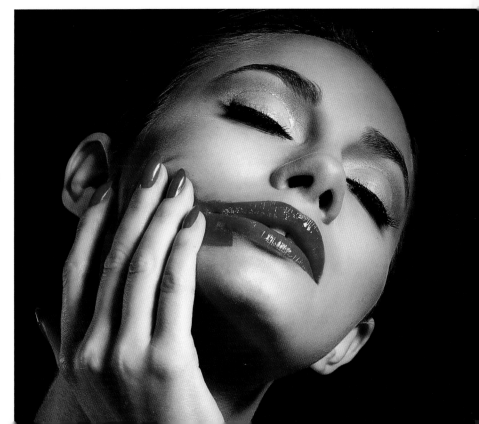

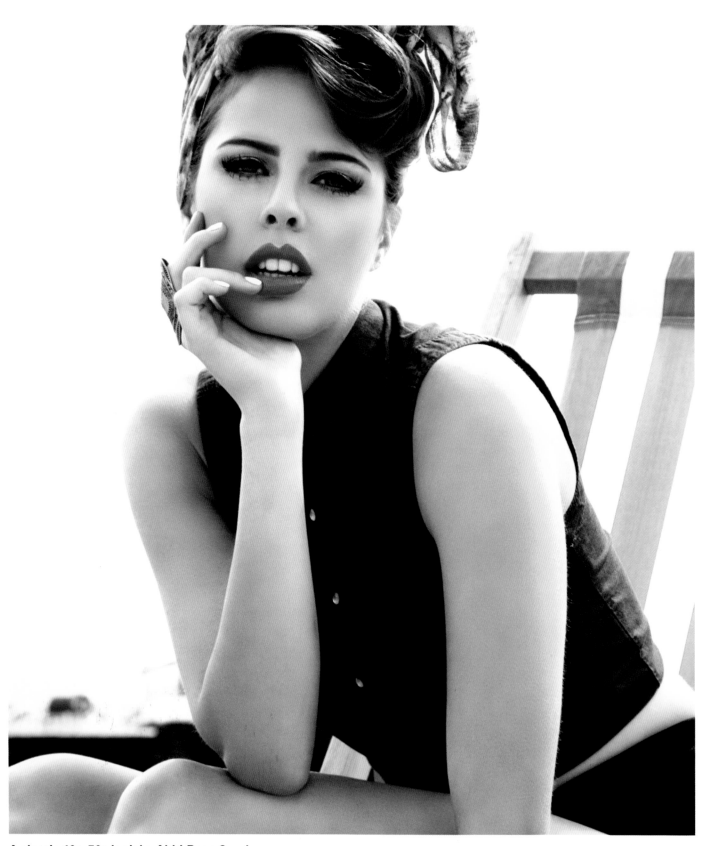

A classic 40s–50s look by Abbi-Rose Crook

Chapter Eight
Vintage Inspiration

From the liner flicks of the 50s to the perfect 40s red lip or pop brights of the 80s, some of the hottest current makeup trends take inspiration from classic vintage looks. Happily, though, flaky rouge and thick pan sticks are things of the past and there are plenty of modern products that can help you put a 21st-century twist on these nostalgic trends.

The 20s was the decade where women really began to experiment with bold makeup. Powdered faces, smoky eyes and defined Cupid's bow pouts were among the iconic looks that defined this era.

As the 30s dawned, so did the Hollywood glamour that would shape the look of the next three decades. While 30s sophistication was all about ivory complexions, and shimmering eyeshadows right up to the pencil-thin brow, the 40s demanded a more practical look for the new wave of women employed to do the jobs of men who had been called up to fight in the war. Makeup was in short supply, forcing women to improvise with substances such as beetroot juice for lipstick and burnt cork for eyeliner. Red lips defined the decade and continued as a trend well into the 50s, where they evolved into orangey hues paired with pale skin, arched brows and the emergence of the liner flick.

The 60s was all about the eyes. Heavy kohl liner and lashings of mascara dominated the baby-doll look, while eyeshadow and lips were kept pale, nude or icy. In the 70s, disco fever brought metallics and the revival of the red lip, also seen in punk later in the decade – think Blondie frontwoman Debbie Harry. Bright colour clashes, heavy stripes of blusher and frosted lipstick defined 80s makeup, while 90s grunge gave us that just-out-of-bed look. The 21st century has seen numerous trends combined with constant flashbacks to the past. The iconic looks will always return, with a modern twist for a new era.

20s cocktail party look

In the 'Roaring Twenties', fashion was completely transformed, with the long hair, modest clothes and minimal makeup of previous decades replaced by shorter, heavily beaded dresses, bobbed hair and strikingly heavy makeup.

Popularized by the flappers, the archetypal 20s look features a strong smoky eye and a rosebud mouth, where the lips are painted with a dark stain in the centre only to create a very rounded pout. The wide eyes and small mouth gave the face a doll-like, heart-shaped finish. For a modern twist on this iconic look, try contouring for a more natural-looking shape. Keeping the lips dark, use shading at the edges and gloss in the centre to give a more subtle result.

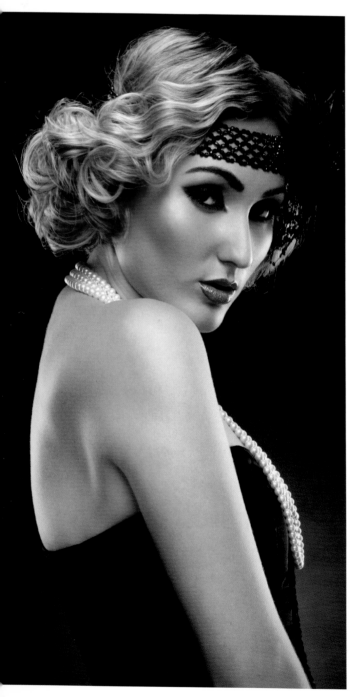

MELANIE DOYLE'S STEP-BY-STEP GUIDE TO THE 20s LOOK WITH A MODERN TWIST

1. Apply an eye primer to the eyelid to make the shadow adhere and last longer. This also helps to intensify colour. Add a light application of primer to the face.

2. Contour using concealer cream. Apply a shade four shades darker than your natural skin tone to the hollows of the cheek and other areas where you want to create a slimming effect. Apply a concealer three shades lighter than your skin to the areas you want to enhance, such as the bridge of the nose, top of the cheekbones and the centre of the forehead. Carefully blend the two colours into the skin with a round, buffing dome-shaped foundation brush.

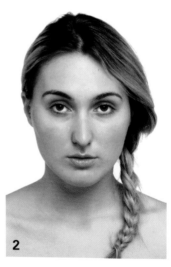

2

3. Apply a liquid foundation mixed with illuminating fluid in the gaps between the highlighter and shader and blend lightly with a dome-shaped brush. Then add a highlighter such as High Beam along the top of the cheekbones.

4. Set makeup with a loose powder then do some additional shading with bronzer to add a little warmth and extra definition to the face, if needed.

5. Define the brows with a matt brow powder, then use a pencil to fill in any gaps and give a more 3D finish.

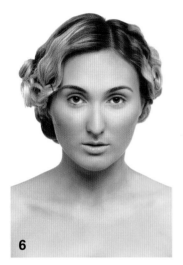

6

6. Add a matt, dark-blue eyeliner to the inner waterline and over the top eyelid and use a small buffing brush to blend, leaving a blurred edge. Then take a sharp, deep purple pencil and draw a line around the inner eye to create a pointed cat's eye. Take the liner from the corner of the outer eye upwards into a wing.

7. Using a flat, square-edged brush, apply a deep violet eyeshadow over the eyelid, up to the socket line and under the lower lashline. Blend towards the crease with a round blending brush to leave a soft outer edge. To keep the strong, winged effect on the outer eye, apply a little more powder with the flat edge of the brush without blending.

8. Curl your lashes then add two sweeps of black mascara before applying a strip eyelash to complete the look.

9. For the lips, apply a creamy violet waterproof liner to the lipline and blend inwards with a small brush. Add a soft pink lip gloss to the centre of both lips and blend out.

10. Apply just a touch of ginger-coloured blusher to the apples of the cheeks and softly blend towards the temples.

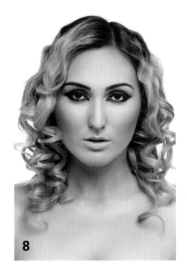

8

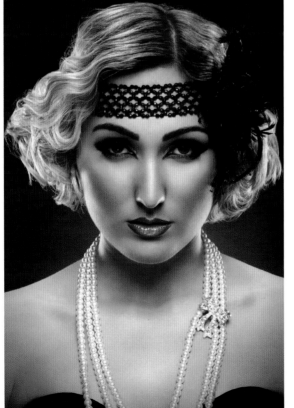

Pro's tips

For the illusion of a fuller pout, apply white shimmer eyeshadow to the centre of the lips. This is a great technique for photoshoots or a big night out to add a little glamour.

*

With strip lashes, apply glue along the lashline and the strip edge with a very fine brush. This ensures a perfect application to last the night.

10

A 20s-inspired look by Melanie Doyle

40s wartime chic

Vintage makeup never goes out of style. The 40s produced another archetypal look – that of wartime women who were encouraged to make do and mend, repurposing lipstick as rouge and charcoal as eyeliner.

In the 40s, makeup trends shifted to a more wholesome look than in the previous two decades, which had favoured exotic icons and dramatic makeup. Many women were going out to work for the first time and makeup needed to be practical. Meanwhile, images of 'Vargas girls', with their hourglass figures, were appearing in magazines such as *Esquire*. These paintings promoted a new ideal of feminine glamour, with bright red lips and pin curls.

Vintage looks are definitely back in vogue, and they don't need much of a modern twist to make a 21st-century statement. For a subtler finish, pick one or two elements from the era, such as a bright lip and defined brow without the liner flick.

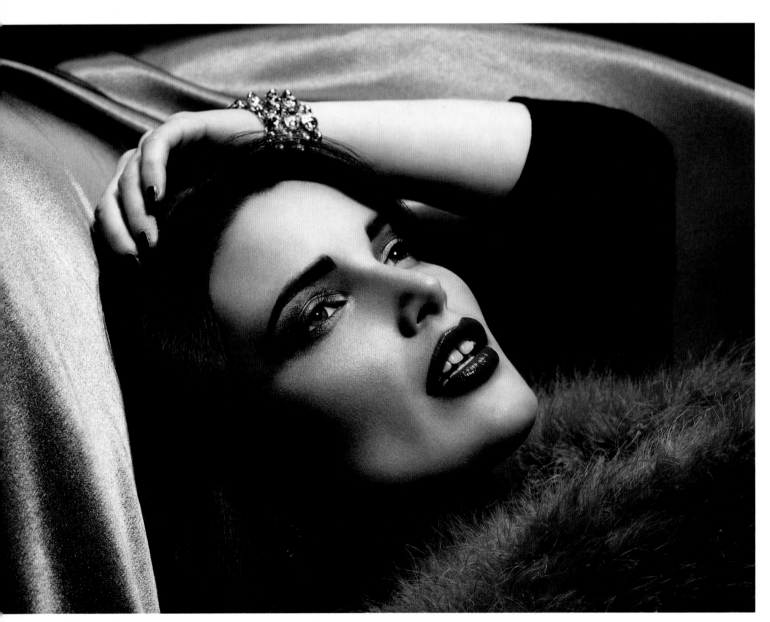

Classic 40s pin up-style makeup by Laura Hunt

LAURA HUNT'S STEP-BY-STEP GUIDE TO A 40s-INSPIRED LOOK

1. Keep the skin tone natural rather than tanned – 40s looks are all about a velvet-textured finish. So, following a natural foundation, use plenty of matt powder.

2. Choose blusher in a natural rose or peach tone. In the 40s, blusher was applied to the apples of the cheeks to create a wholesome look. Always use powder rather than cream blush, applying with a blusher brush in a swirling motion.

3. Sweep a natural and feminine-toned eyeshadow, such as a soft lavender or pink, across the eyelid. Then define the eye by applying a darker but still neutral shade, such as brown or muted grey, into the socket line.

4. Take a gel or liquid liner along the upper lashline and finish in a flick. In the 40s, women wore more liquid eyeliner than women in the 20s or 30s. However, the flick shouldn't be as accentuated as it became in the 50s.

5. Apply black or brown mascara to accentuate the eye.

6. Brows were well groomed. Brush them through then add a little brow pencil in light strokes, keeping the natural shape.

7. Use an orange-based red on the lips, starting with a lipliner to create a natural but full shape; then fill with a matching lipstick. Blot, reapply and set with powder.

8. Finally, paint your nails to match your lip colour. This was an essential part of 40s and 50s looks, influenced by Revlon's 'matching lips and fingertips' ad campaigns.

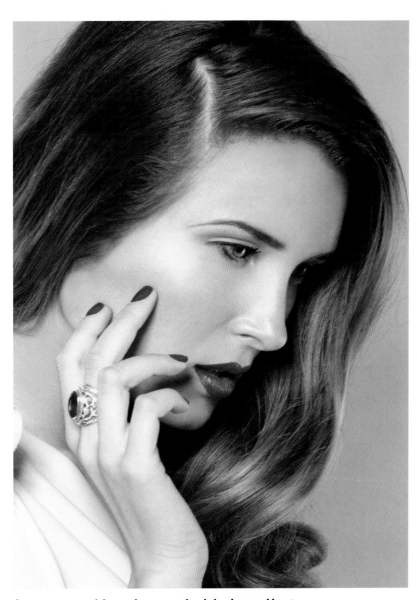

A more wearable and current look by Laura Hunt, influenced by 40s trends

PROFILE
LAURA HUNT

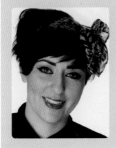

Laura Hunt is a freelance MUA. She runs her own vintage hair and makeup events team called The Beauty Queens with hair and makeup pro Gina Dowle. Laura also works in fashion, advertising, music and TV and has been involved in commercials for brands such as Adidas and Starbucks.

50s siren

Once the war was over, makeup became more glamorous. Influenced by Hollywood stars and pin-ups, women went for the ultra-feminine look and took their time applying makeup. Modern-day sirens such as Dita Von Teese and Kelly Brook take their cue from 50s femininity, sporting bright red lipstick and pairing it with an accentuated eyeliner flick.

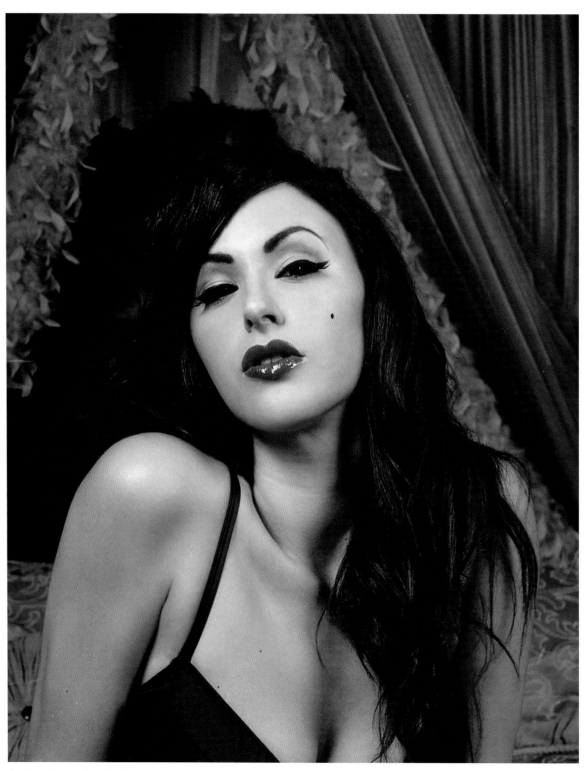

A classic 50s look, given a modern burlesque edge by Laura Hunt

LAURA HUNT'S STEP-BY-STEP GUIDE TO A 50s SIREN LOOK

1. As in the 40s, 50s women kept their skin natural in tone and matt or velvet in finish. Use a soft, fine powder foundation applied with a large powder brush to create this effect.

2. Blusher was applied along the cheekbones and to the apples of the cheeks for a more glamorous effect. To get the look, use a powder blush in a rose, coral or peach tone.

3. For the eyes, choose a flat, ivory shadow, without any shimmer, and apply it across the whole of the lid using a shadow brush, then use a neutral colour such as soft taupe to define the socket line.

4. Winged eyeliner is probably the most important step in your 50s-inspired look. There was a preference for a heavier, more extenuated flick than in the 40s, so use a liquid liner and go thicker than you normally would, finishing in a long flick.

5. Apply mascara, then add false lashes. These became very popular in the 1950s. Choose a dramatic, long length and apply using fine tweezers, starting at the inner corner of the eye.

6. Brows should be thick, dark and highly arched, with a squarer finish than in the 40s. Try using a brow stencil with a powder slightly darker than your natural brow. Stipple the colour in with a brow brush and set with brow gel.

7. Use a blue-red lipliner and lipstick to achieve a full finish, then coat with a clear gloss for the ultimate siren pout.

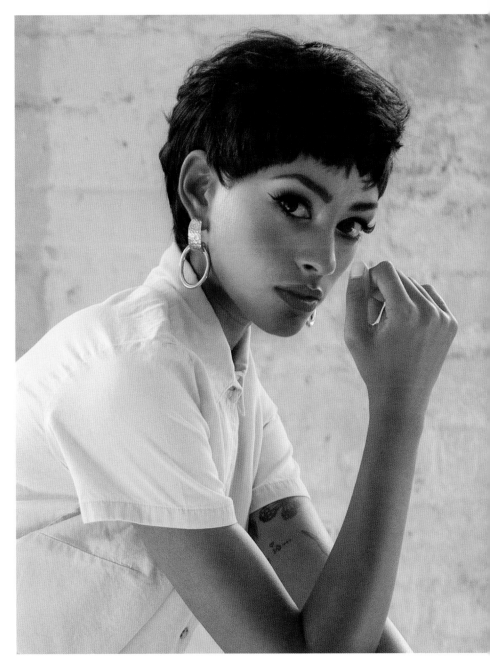

The opposite of siren, but with similar makeup, the gamine look was inspired by the actress Audrey Hepburn. This modern take on the 50s waif is by Laura Hunt.

60s mod

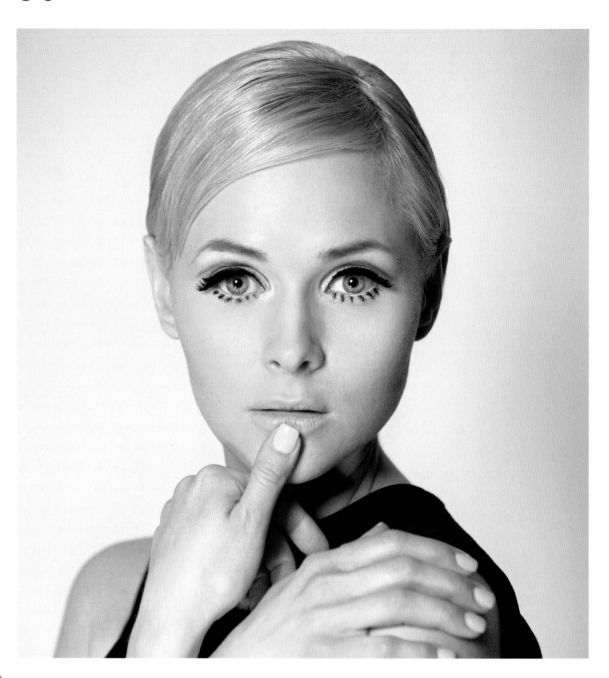

Pro's tip

To maintain that 60s vibe, keep the sooty eyes the main focus, but try grey liner and clumpy lashes for daytime. This looks super cute with pale lips and summer skin.

While the mid-60s brought a back-to-nature, makeup-free look associated with the hippie movement, the most iconic 60s look is that of the black, sooty eyes and pale nude lips modelled by Twiggy. This mod makeup look was big in the early part of the decade and was all about making eyes the standout feature. Keep everything matt and go monochrome for a look that still screams high fashion in the 21st century.

DENISE RABOR'S STEP-BY-STEP GUIDE TO THE 60s-INSPIRED MOD LOOK

1. Skin should be velvety – use a foundation with a matt or natural finish so that you don't have to use much powder. Blush is fairly low key so choose a shade with a soft, tawny peach tone for pale skin types or a warm brown or orange colour for darker skins.

2. Eyebrows should be groomed, but still natural-looking, so resist the urge to overdraw them. Try an eyeshadow primer to help your eye makeup last longer and prevent smudging.

3. Take a white or cream eyeshadow and apply it over your entire eyelid, blending outwards. Then apply a grey, black or dark brown matt shadow to the crease of your eye using either a socket brush or an angled eyeshadow brush. Blend so you don't have a hard line, just a shadowed crease.

4. Add black liner along the upper lashline. The 60s look was all about a matt finish so try a gel liner rather than a glossy liquid and gently blend at the edges.

5. Curl your lashes, then apply two coats of black volumizing mascara to both top and bottom lashes. Alternatively, apply false lashes, but make sure they are not too long or feline in style; the idea is to look wide-eyed.

6. The eyes are very much the focus of this look, so ideally your lips should be kept neutral with either a gloss or a flesh-toned matt lipstick.

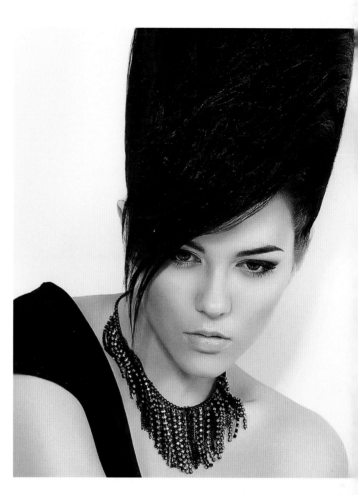

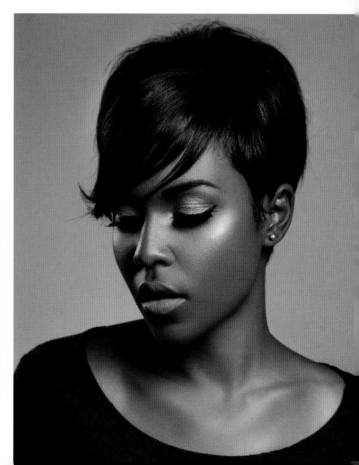

PROFILE
DENISE RABOR

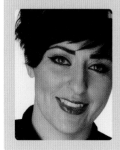

Denise Rabor's work has appeared in *Harper's Bazaar*, *Vogue*, *Elle*, *Vanity Fair* and many other magazines. She produces her own online makeup, skincare and wellness magazine, *Wow Beauty*. She loves the diversity of the beauty industry and working with women of all ages and ethnicities.

70s disco diva

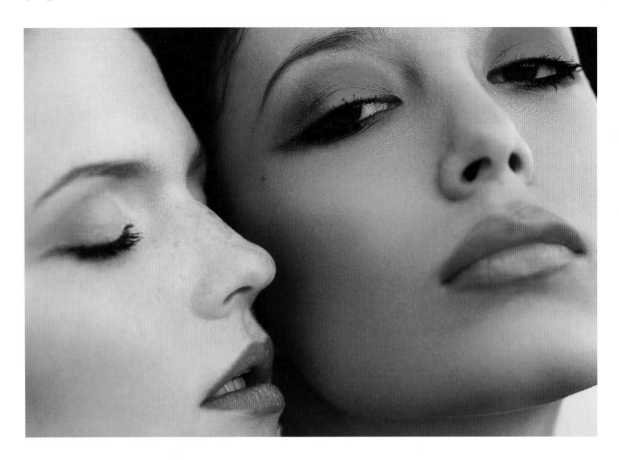

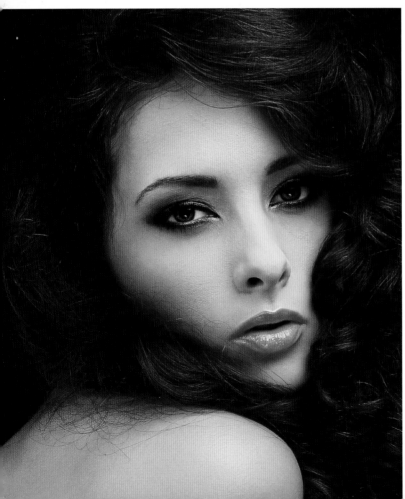

The 1970s brought a dichotomy in makeup, with the natural, barely there hippie look of the 60s still a major influence. At the other end of the scale, glitters and metallics were taken to the extreme in disco culture. Blue eyeshadows and bright pink blush gave a striking femininity to 70s looks on and off the dance floor.

For a modern twist, try using blue as an accent colour on a metallic silver eye. Or use colour over the lid only, and pair with brushed-up brows to bring the look into the 21st century. 'People are scared of blue, but you can bring it back in subtle ways; it doesn't have to be Abba style,' says pro MUA Anne Bowcock. 'The look I created [see facing page] was extreme, for a high-impact photo shoot, but you can play it down and add black liner and mascara for a more wearable look.'

If you don't feel comfortable with loud colours, trying mixing a small amount of blue eyeshadow with a metallic silver shadow for a paler finish. Pat it all over the eyelid and buff the edges to soften, then apply a thin line below the bottom lid – disco eyes are about all-around colour. Dab a lighter colour in the centre of the lid and the inner corners of the eyes to give a 3D finish.

ANNE BOWCOCK'S STEP-BY-STEP GUIDE TO A 70s DISCO DIVA LOOK

1. For this look I started with a nice luminous Illamasqua base, then added a small amount of pink blusher to bring some glow. Don't do heavy contouring as you want the look to be all about the eyes.

2. Prep the eyes with primer, then use a cream blue shadow right up to the brow and below the lower lashline to three-quarters of the way in. Set with a blue powder shadow.

3. Do the same with green cream then powder shadow along the browbone.

4. Use a highlighter along the inner quarter of the lower lashline and around the eye up to meet the blue.

5. I finished the look with green mascara, then used some brow powder to define the brows before brushing them up and setting them with clear gel.

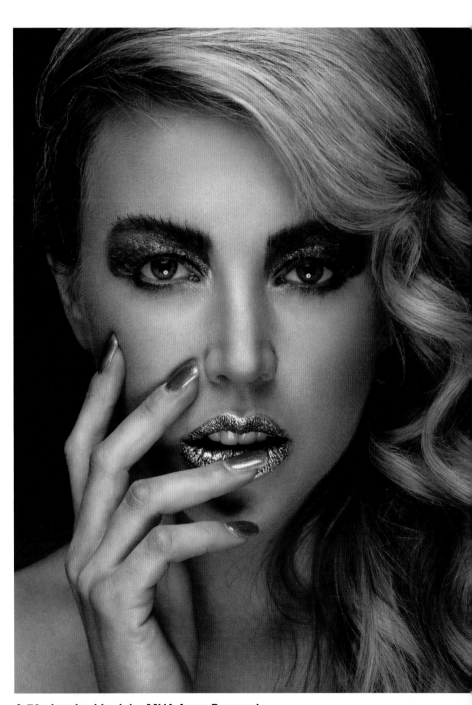

Disco tips

For a more modern look, don't take the blue shadow up to the browbone, just place it over the lid then bring some green shadow into the inner corner and blend.

*

You could add some coordinating glitter to make the eyes sparkle. Put a bit of glitter gel on the back of your hand, dip a fine brush into it and then into your glitter. Place it carefully along the lashline, then along the crease line of the eye.

Add false lashes to break up the colour, and set with black liquid eyeliner.

A 70s-inspired look by MUA Anne Bowcock

80s brights

Bold colours defined 80s makeup, from clashing brights worn by pop stars such as Madonna and Cyndi Lauper to the stripes of blusher and bold lips sported by the yuppie brigade. Teamed with big hair, huge shoulder-pads and plenty of bling, 80s faces were about overstatement.

While neon pink blushers and colour clashing may have been left in the past, there are plenty of ways to bring 80s brights into the 21st century. Start by choosing one feature, usually the eyes or the lips, and keep it powdery and matt to make the colour really pop.

Vintage inspiration

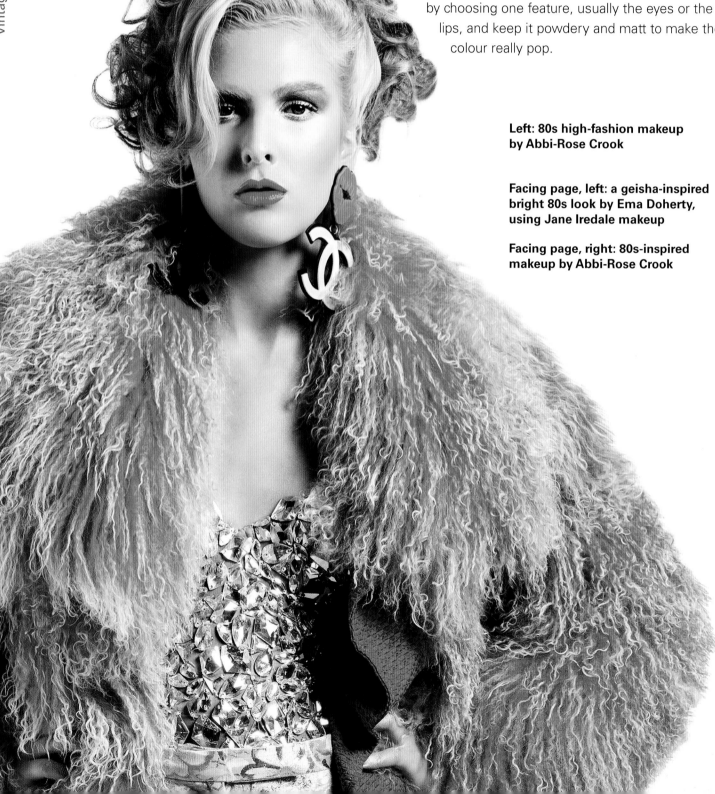

Left: 80s high-fashion makeup by Abbi-Rose Crook

Facing page, left: a geisha-inspired bright 80s look by Ema Doherty, using Jane Iredale makeup

Facing page, right: 80s-inspired makeup by Abbi-Rose Crook

EMA DOHERTY'S TIPS FOR USING BRIGHTS

- If you use just one bright shade, it can be reflected as an accent in different areas of the face. If using more than one bright colour, then apply each in just one area otherwise the look can become too busy and the bold statement will be lost.

- Bright and neon colours look bolder if they are matt. Pearly or shimmery tones reflect too much light, so sharpness is lost.

- Brights have the advantage of being suitable for both shading and highlighting an area, so choose where you place them carefully.

- Use cosmetics with high pigment so that the payoff of colour is strong and quick to build. If necessary, wet the powder to get a concentrated effect.

- To give brightness to an otherwise mid or duller tone, use a matt white eye pencil underneath the colour to lift it.

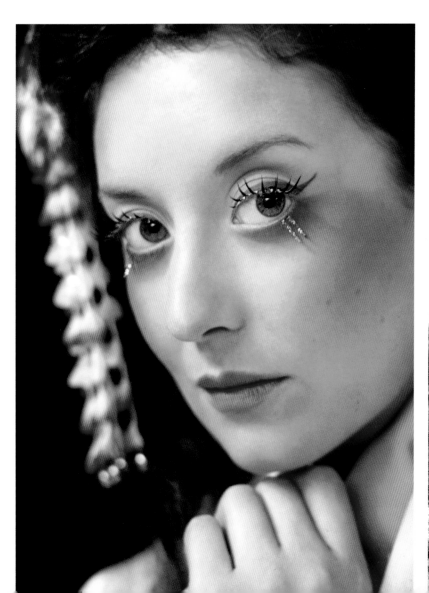
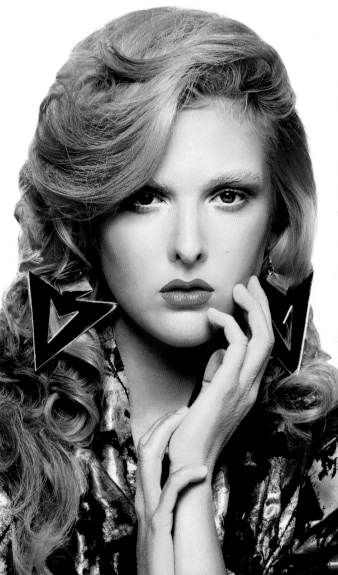

Picture credits and acknowledgments

Picture credits

Title page: hair and makeup: Pamela Moss; photographer: David Slater; model: Julie Burville

Contents page: makeup and nails: Abbi-Rose Crook; model: Charlotte Girdwood; photography: Leighton Parry; styling and hair: Joey Bevan

Page 6: makeup: Melanie Brown; photographer: Tory Smith, www.tory-smith.com; photo assistant: Sanna Halmekoski; hair stylist: KT Gallagher; stylist: Emma Lightbown; nail artist: Diana Drummond; model: Loredana @ M&P

Page 7: makeup: Abbi-Rose Crook; photography: Jayesh Pankhania @ SixtyOne Productions; hair: Carmen Amelia; model: Olga @ M+P; retouching: Pratik Naik of Solstice Retouch

Page 8: makeup: Tamara Tott; photographer: Dany Baldwin; hair: Roy Hayward; styling: Christina Davydova

Page 27: makeup: Jen Hunter; photography: Take A Shot Photography; model: Karen Montague

Page 30: image, top: from a shoot for Sassi Holford London; makeup: Sarah Brock; photography: Simon Powell

Page 30: image, bottom: from a shoot for Philippa Lepley; makeup: Sarah Brock; photography: Nicole Nodland

Page 31: makeup: Sarah Brock; photography: Anthony Edwin

Page 33: makeup: Catherine Bailey; photography: www.zanephoto.com

Page 34: image from a shoot for Bare Minerals; makeup: Sarah Jane Froom

Page 36: image from a shoot for Sothys

Pages 40–41: makeup: Jen Hunter; photography: Take A Shot Photography; model Karen Montague

Page 43: image from a shoot for Sothys

Page 45: makeup: Salina Thind

Page 47: image, top: makeup: Ema Doherty

Page 48: images, top and bottom: makeup: Tamara Tott

Page 49: images, top left, bottom left and bottom right: makeup: Tamara Tott

Page 51: image, top left: makeup: Daniel Sandler

Page 54: images from a shoot for HD Brows; brows by Nilam Holmes-Patel

Page 56: profile image of Armand Beasley: photographer: Adam Yate

Page 62: image from a shoot for Harlem Carter; makeup: Anne Bowcock; makeup assistant: Shannon Keegan; photographer: William Clark; hair and model: Michelle Jo-an Hodson

Page 66: image, bottom: from a shoot for Sothys

Page 70: makeup: Jen Hunter; photography: Take A Shot Photography; hair: Harriet Newton; model: Rosanna Marie Owen

Pages 72: images, bottom: products from the Make-up by HD Brows range

Page 73: images: products from the Make-up by HD Brows range

Page 74: makeup: Catherine Bailey; photography: www.twistyimages.com

Page 76: hair and makeup: Pamela Moss; photography: Darren Shaw; model: Charlie Long

Page 77: hair and makeup: Pamela Moss; photography: Darren Shaw; model: Katy Pullinger

Page 78–9: makeup: Tamara Tott

Page 82: makeup and design: Anne Bowcock; photographer: William Clark; model: Jenna Lee White; hair and design: Michelle Jo-an Hudson; makeup assistant: Sarah Allan

Page 89: makeup: Kirstie Bower using Mii Cosmetics; model: Taylar Leake

Page 93: makeup: Jen Hunter; photography: Take A Shot Photography; hair: Harriet Newton; model: Bethany Cammack

Page 94: makeup, hair and styling: Alyn Waterman; photographer: Helen Joseph Photography; headdress: Verdure Floral Design; model: Luisa Hayden

Page 95: image, top: makeup, hair and styling: Alyn Waterman; photographer: Helen Joseph Photography; headdress: Verdure Floral Design;

model: Luisa Hayden; image, bottom: makeup and hair by Alyn Waterman; photographer: Helen Joseph Photography; model: Anisa Akram

Page 96–7: makeup and hair: Alyn Waterman; photographer: Helen Joseph Photography; model: Anisa Akram

Page 98: makeup: Abbi-Rose Crook; photographer: Leighton Parry; styling and hair: Joey Bevan; model: Courtney King

Page 103: makeup: Abbi-Rose Crook; photography: Jayesh Pankhania @ SixtyOne Productions; hair: Carmen Amelia; model: Olga @ M+P; retouching: Pratik Naik of Solstice Retouch

Page 104: makeup and hair: Abbi-Rose Crook; photography: Harley Moon Kemp

Page 105: makeup: Abbi-Rose Crook; styling and hair: Joey Bevan; photographer: Leighton Parry; model: Courtney King

Page 106: image, top: hair and makeup: Pamela Moss; photographer: David Slater; model: Julie Burville

Page 107: makeup: Jo Coletta; photography: Shooting Beauty Production

Page 107, bottom: makeup: Abbi-Rose Crook; photographer: Leighton Parry; styling and hair: Joey Bevan; models: Kylie Van Beek and Laura Hurtado

Page 108: makeup: Abbi-Rose Crook; photography: Jayesh Pankhania @ SixtyOne Productions; hair: Carmen Amelia; model: Olga @ M+P; retouching: Pratik Naik of Solstice Retouch

Page 109: makeup and nail: Abbi-Rose Crook using Facelace; model: Eva @ Sapphires; photography: Condry Calvin Milo; hair: Joey Bevan

Page 112: make-up: Abbi-Rose Crook; hair: Kasia Fortuna; photographer: Ruth Rose; assistant: Katie Jane Mabey; stylist: Steph Colaco; model: Sylwia at First; digital imaging: Ben Secret

Page 114–15: makeup: Melanie Doyle;

photographer: Ian McManus; model: Claudia Frances

Page 116: makeup: Laura Hunt; photographer: Dominic Nicholls

Page 117: makeup: Laura Hunt; photographer: Sarah Louise Johnson; hair: Eugene Davis; model: Dite

Page 118: hair and makeup: Laura Hunt; photographer: Nathan Atia; model: Nina Hearne

Page 119: makeup: Laura Hunt; photographer: Katy Winterflood; hair: Eugene Davis

Page 123: makeup and design: Anne Bowcock; photographer: William Clark; model: Jenna Lee White; hair and design: Michelle Jo-an Hudson; makeup assistant: Sarah Allan

Page 124: makeup: Abbi-Rose Crook; model agency: PRM; photography: Chris Lord; styling and hair: Joey Bevan

Page 125: image, left: makeup and hair: Ema Doherty

Page 125: image, right: makeup and hair: Laura Hunt; photographer: Nathan Atia; model: Nina Hearne

Acknowledgments

With thanks to all the amazing makeup artists who shared their time and talents to make this book possible, particularly Alyn Waterman and Abbi-Rose Crook for their guidance. Thanks also to the following for their help and support: Matt Wilkinson, Tory Smith, Stefania Crockett, Mary-Tabitha Wilkin, Anna Hirsch, Emma Rowbottom, Gosia Krajewski, Jacki Wadeson, Faye Yarnall, Nadine Attar, Joelle Pugh, Lindsay Stewart, Lorien Norden, Kayleigh Kniveton, Cat Halliwell and Emily Wood.

Stockists

ARTDECO www.artdeco.com

Bare Minerals www.bareminerals.co.uk

BECCA www.beccacosmetics.com

Benefit Cosmetics www.benefitcosmetics.com

Bobbi Brown Cosmetics www.bobbibrowncosmetics.com

Bourjois www.bourjois.com

Chanel www.chanel.com/makeup

Clarins www.groupeclarins.com

Clinique www.clinique.com

Corn Silk Powder www.boots.com

Cosmetics à la carte www.alacartelondon.com

Daniel Sandler Makeup danielsandler.com

Dermalogica www.dermalogica.com

DHC www.dhccare.com

Elemis www.elemis.com

Environ www.environ.co.za / www.iiaa.eu

Eye Rock www.rockbeautylondon.com

Face Lace www.face-lace.com

Giorgio Armani www.armanibeauty.com

Guinot guinot.com

HD Brows http://hdbrows.com

Hourglass www.hourglasscosmetics.com

Illamasqua www.illamasqua.com

Jane Iredale http://janeiredale.com

Joan Collins Timeless Beauty www.joancollinsbeauty.com

Kiehl's www.kiehls.com

Le Maq Pro lemaqpro.com

Lily Lolo www.lilylolo.co.uk

Liz Earle uk.lizearle.com

MAC www.maccosmetics.com

Make Up by HD Brows hdbrows.com

MaskerAide www.maskeraide.com

Mii www.miicosmetics.com

Murad www.murad.com

NARS www.narscosmetics.com

Revlon www.revlon.com

Rimmel www.rimmellondon.com

RMK www.rmkrmk.com

Royal & Langnickel www.royalbrush.com

Sensibio www.bioderma.com

Skindinavia http://skindinavia.com

Skyn Iceland www.skyniceland.com

Smashbox www.smashbox.com

Sothys www.sothys.com

Stage Line Professional www.stagelineprofessional.com

Stila www.stilacosmetics.com

Urban Decay www.urbandecay.com

Youngblood http://ybskin.co.uk